Living Life
Lean

A Practical Guide to Achieving and
Maintaining a Healthy Weight

BRUCE E. MORGAN, MS, ATC

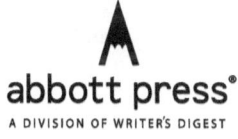

abbott press®

A DIVISION OF WRITER'S DIGEST

Abbott Press books may be ordered through booksellers or by contacting:

Abbott Press
1663 Liberty Drive
Bloomington, IN 47403
www.abbottpress.com
Phone: 1-866-697-5310

Because of the dynamic nature of the Internet, any web addresses or
links contained in this book may have changed since publication and
may no longer be valid. The views expressed in this work are solely those
of the author and do not necessarily reflect the views of the publisher,
and the publisher hereby disclaims any responsibility for them.

Any people depicted in stock imagery provided by Thinkstock are models,
and such images are being used for illustrative purposes only.
Certain stock imagery © Thinkstock.

ISBN: 978-1-4582-1251-1 (sc)
ISBN: 978-1-4582-1252-8 (hc)
ISBN: 978-1-4582-1253-5 (e)

Library of Congress Control Number: 2013920381

Printed in the United States of America.

Abbott Press rev. date: 12/13/2013

To those who have tried and failed,
yet in whom the desire to live life lean continues
to burn brightly, this book is dedicated.

"*Success is the child of drudgery and perseverance. It cannot be coaxed or bribed; pay the price and it is yours.*"

– Orison Sweet Marden

Contents

Acknowledgements

Throughout the process of writing this book, I have sought the counsel and kind assistance of friends and colleagues alike. They have unselfishly given their time and expertise, which in no small way has contributed to bringing this project to fruition. To all of you who, through either word or deed, have participated in the process, please accept my most humble and sincere thanks.

Preface

Enter *weight loss* into a book search at Amazon.com and you'll discover over 80,000 titles exploring the subject available for purchase. Assuming for a moment that you had no prior knowledge of the subject, you could infer from that number alone that weight loss was either popular, controversial or both, and that about it multiple opinions existed. On all accounts, you would of course be correct. Weight loss unites us in our desire to achieve it and our failure to understand it. Compounding this failure to understand is the chaos and confusion that grows out of the din of voices, each summoning up their own science to support their opinions. Through their books and websites, they offer new or unique, but always better than those that preceded it, methods to melt away the fat and reveal the you that you had always hoped to be. Thinking that they will deliver on their promise, you turn to first one, and then another, and then still others, imagining that this will be the one that leaves others gawking at you in admiration.

Our popular culture assaults us with images of lean women and chiseled men who serve to shape our perception of what is normal or desirable. So distorted is the lens through which we view such things that in the Hollywood of today Marilyn Monroe and Jane Russell, the screen sirens of their day, might struggle to find work.

More fleshy still were the women portrayed and glorified by the seventeenth century Flemish painter Peter Paul Rubens. In an era when being full of figure was thought to be a sign of wealth and privilege, Rubens' work cast *them* as the ideal. So synonymous with the plus-sized female figure is Rubens that nearly four hundred years after his death women of generous proportion continue to be referred to as "Rubenesque".

My point is that as times change, so too do our perceptions and preferences. Regardless how a particular group or era describes their ideal, the norm generally lies somewhere outside of it. By its very definition, the norm tends to be a typical or representative value that clusters around the midpoint of a group of data. As such, whatever the public perception may be, we middling Americans are the present norm. Those actors featured in our movies and TV programs are not the norm, they may be the modern day ideal, but the norm they are not. In fact, in terms of their weight, they may be two standard deviations to the left of the norm.

The new norm I'm sad to say is twenty-five pounds heavier than the norm of 1960 (for both men and women age 20-74). Lest you think the twenty-five pounds is all muscle think again. Occurring along with this weight gain are increases in body mass index that today come dangerously close to what would be judged the lower ranges of obesity.

Taken together, today we are confronted with a two-pronged problem: the first is related to how we perceive and define the ideal where our physical form is concerned, and the second is connected to how far from that ideal the vast majority of us are. With respect to both, we should work to come to some middle ground. Lose weight? Yes! Lose weight to achieve a societally determined ideal? No! Better, I think, we should reexamine what we as a society deem to be ideal. Failing that, then each of us individually must redefine it for ourselves. It is right and proper that you work to reduce your body fat stores. Whatever else they may be, these fat stores impede your vitality, adversely affect your self-perception and put you at increased risk of chronic illness. For these reasons and others, decreasing the amount of fat you carry is to your benefit.

Within these pages, you will find no simple solutions, no quick fixes, and no amazing new science that promises to melt away your unwanted fat. Neither will you find six-minute body shaping workout routines nor recipes that purport to burn fat. Instead, what you will receive are the brass tacks of weight loss, the plain, simple and unvarnished truth. It is with this in mind that I ask you to remove your rose colored glasses before you turn to the next page because from that page forward I will not attempt to deceive you into believing that weight loss is child's play. In fact, my mantra will be that weight loss is a difficult and frustrating process. My purpose for saying so will not be to crush your spirit, but rather to support you during those times when you imagine that only you struggle to achieve your weight loss goals. Were that true, then eighty thousand plus books revolving around weight loss would not be in print and more than two hundred million Americans would not be overweight or obese.

If you are one among those two hundred million, know that there is hope for you. If you have tried to lose weight in the past and failed, or if you have succeeded in the short-term only to regain the weight some months later, do not accept carrying that weight as your final fate. It is possible to amend your lifestyle in order to bring about sustainable weight loss. The steps toward achieving that end I present for you here. Go confidently into your journey, the rewards of increased health, stamina and self-esteem await you.

Chapter 1

More Isn't Always Better

America is a land of many riches; those of us who call it home are, to my thinking, fortunate to be able to do so. Geopolitical strife aside, America still offers the greatest opportunities for growth and prosperity. It is principally for this reason that those who seek better lives for themselves and their families aspire to settle here. Since our founding it has always been so.

The opportunities about which I speak are not purely financial. While it is true that the American standard of living is among the highest in the world, it is, I suspect, the freedoms that our society affords that make life here such an attractive notion.

I can't know what impressions our country leaves upon those who visit here or upon those who arrive here to begin their lives anew, but it has occurred to me throughout the course of my travels to distant countries that those who come here must be struck by our abundance. The particular abundance may vary dependent upon the proclivity of the observer, but that which must be especially awe-inspiring is the variety and sheer volume of our food choices. Surely we are not alone in that regard; other countries share our good fortune as it relates to the availability of foodstuffs, but few countries can boast of the vast repositories (let's call them grocery stores) where these items are held for inspection, and ultimately, purchase.

Far from boasting about such repositories, other countries are likely to point to them as a symptom of the disease that has taken hold of our country and threatens to shake it to its very foundation. As I sit here and peck away at my keyboard, fully two-thirds of my fellow Americans are either overweight or obese. The statistics related to this epidemic are truly staggering, both in terms of the increases in the rates during the course of the past few decades and the costs that our society must bear to manage the medical issues that grow out of this alarming shift in the direction of obesity.

Let me assure you that I, as much as anyone, know that none of us gets out of this alive. We will all one-day breathe our last. That being so, some might argue that they should be left to lead the lives they choose. Forgetting the cost that each of us are made to pay to care for those whose choices lead to protracted illness and non-productivity, it is my general feeling that they should be free to do as they will. I do not attempt to reach those through this book. After all, we cannot, in spite of Mayor Bloomberg's (New York City, 2002-2013) attempts to do so, legislate good health. Neither can we bully people into it, although Jillian Michaels has made millions trying to do just that. People must go willingly into this challenge, not poked or prodded but self-motivated. I address those people who hope to maximize their lives if not extend them outright, those who look to reduce the weight that they feel limits their opportunities to enjoy their lives to the fullest. For those there is a path that leads to increased vigor and restored health. Mind you, for most it will be a long and difficult slog. But as is true with most of life's battles, those that are hard-won are most treasured.

This particular path begins with one especially agonizing first step, a step that comes in the form of an admission: the weight you carry is a product of your own doing. As a younger person, I attempted to convey this very message to a group of "weight-challenged" women in Northern California. Were it not for some apologetic backpedalling, they would have run me out of town on a rail. Vowing to fight another day I revisit that notion here.

For entirely too long we have been told that our problems, whatever they might be, are not of our own creation. We are all victims of outside forces that conspire to separate us from our bliss, or so we are led to believe. As it pertains to our weight, we cannot break free from the legacy bequeathed to us by our parents and theirs. Or can we? Sure, some inescapable genetic predispositions dictate where and how we store our excess body fat. However, for the excess fat itself, we must take responsibility. Some might find this stance a bit harsh, particularly for those who began adding to their fat stores at a very early age. Still, it is my feeling that we must own our weight if we are going to own the changes that ultimately bring our weight under control. Sadly, that alone will not get you to where you want to be. Others have accepted that responsibility and failed to achieve their goal. In fact, the diet landscape is awash with such failure. How then are we, they, any of us to succeed when failure is so commonplace? I'll tell you what, let's come back to success after we've had a good hard look at failure.

Most of you who have bothered to read this far have at one time or another participated in a diet program. In fact, statistics indicate that many of you have involved yourselves in multiple such programs. Encouraged by a friend or family member who saw the diet featured on *Dr. Oz*, or read it was used to great success by a long list of Hollywood celebrities, you thought, why not? Spurred on by draconian calorie restriction, you might even have appreciated some early weight loss. But overtime you simply could not adhere to the diet's narrow and/or stringent guidelines and back came the weight. This same scenario plays out in American homes on a daily basis. Whatever the plan, whichever foods it vilifies, and however it purports to accomplish its purposes, most diets fail.

While the reasons for these failures may be many, the common thread that seems to run through all diets is their failure to address what I consider our pathologic relationship with food. We Americans eat for reasons other than to satisfy hunger. If only hunger drove our desire to eat, none of us would be overweight, let alone obese. And if hunger motivated us to eat, then it stands to reason that satisfying hunger would cause us to cease eating. Sadly for many, hunger is but one of a litany of reasons that compel us to feed. Equally sad is the fact that satisfying our hunger fails to turn off the need to feed. Thanksgiving dinner is not the only meal that leaves us feeling discontentedly overindulged. Yet in this pattern we persist. Eating not necessarily because we're hungry, but because we're angry, or frustrated, or lonely, or disappointed, or unloved, or bored, or because someone else is eating, or because it's time to eat, or because there is food to eat, or we have an event to celebrate, or one to mourn. Food is our friend that accompanies us through good times and bad, and provides us with comfort from the rigors and stresses of the outside world. Food is a palliative, a band-aid covering the wounds inflicted by the lives we lead. Food does these things and at no time in the process does it judge us for our choices.

Making matters worse is our predilection to consume alcohol. A palliative in its own right, alcohol is the great disinhibitor. Consumed in the proper quantities, it removes the restraints that might otherwise influence, if not govern our decision-making. Here I speak with specific reference to eating, but as we're all aware, alcohol and its mind-altering cousins can and do affect our ability to make reasoned decisions in all manner of subject areas.

Perhaps if it provided some nutritional value I might be more forgiving of alcohol. Aside from some speculative benefit tied to tannins found in red wine, I think one would be hard pressed to make a compelling argument in favor of its regular consumption. So regular is some people's alcohol consumption, that if asked the question, "When did you have your last drink?", they are more likely to refer to a clock than a calendar. For any number of reasons, our weight included, consuming alcohol on such a frequent basis is a practice that we simply cannot sustain.

As a rule, I discourage folks from drinking their calories. Regardless their source, but particularly alcohol, beverages tend to be high in calories and low in nutrient density. For those unfamiliar with the term, nutrient density speaks to the relationship between the nutritional value of a food and its caloric content. A food is said to be nutrient dense if it delivers high concentrations of vitamins and minerals with a low calorie cost. Still not clear? A good example would be a comparison between whole milk and nonfat or skim milk. Along with its fat, skim milk has more than 50 percent of its calories removed when compared with whole milk. With its nutrient profile otherwise unaffected, skim milk would be considered more nutrient dense than whole milk would. Similarly, grilled chicken rates higher in its nutrient density than the Colonel's breaded and fried alternative does. Perhaps an arcane concept, but I believe it is critical to the discussion and because it will be revisited later I want to be certain it is well understood.

I trust it is also understood that we Americans need to come to terms with our issues surrounding food. Is there a heretofore-undiscovered biologic imperative that drives the human feeding behavior, or are we simply sublimating eating for our feelings of hostility, anger, isolation, frustration, (you fill in the blank)? An appropriate, although at first blush bizarre, follow-up question might be, in the way we eat are we more akin to dogs or cats? As a dog lover and one who has had a long-standing antipathy for cats, it grieves me to acknowledge that, at least as it concerns how each manages their food, cats are superior. While dogs typically wolf down their meals then rush to sit alongside the family dinner table in hopes of earning a scrap, cats cannot be bothered. Cats eat when the mood strikes and even then only in moderation. Cats seem to understand that when they finish their food, more will appear in its place. Dogs, on the other hand, eat everything placed before them and then quickly set out in pursuit of something more. Dogs seem to operate with the belief that they'd better eat now, for the future is uncertain.

Sure our futures may be uncertain, but most of us have never known true hunger; a meal, or at the very least a snack, is always in the near offing. It is not necessary for us to behave like dogs and eat as if there will be no tomorrow. In the case of our diets, if nothing else, cats can teach us a lesson - moderation is the key.

Beyond that one lesson, and regardless of how much we may love our pets they are not we, and we are not they. We occupy a unique niche in the animal kingdom. Although we don't always live up to our billing, humans are meant to be reasonable and rational, problem solvers of the highest order, capable of unraveling the mysteries of life, but yet unable to achieve or sustain weight loss. It is with that as a backdrop that those who pedal diet programs are able to convince America's overweight population that weight loss is tantamount to splitting the atom in terms of difficulty. From the perspective of those who struggle to achieve weight loss, the belief there is something more at work here than simple calorie restriction seems reasonable. The presence of certain disease states, the taking of a variety of medications, even a dysfunctional hypothalamus or thyroid *might* be factors for weight gain, but the truth is that such factors intervene rather infrequently. Similarly cited is the go-to nutritional issue du jour - gluten sensitivity. Many are touting it as a factor contributing to weight gain, but the corroborating evidence is scant. For most, the difficulty arises from the inability to accurately estimate the number of calories consumed as a function of the confusion over serving size. Our weight has increased in direct proportion with our meal sizes, and this is no coincidence. Much has been made of portion size today versus that of years ago. Today, large quantities of inexpensive items (what I refer to as "brown foods"), everything from pizza to bagels to burgers and fries, have morphed into supersized versions of their former selves and altered our perception of what a meal should look like.

With the changes in the portion sizes of our food come changes to the sizes of the plates, bowls, and cups in which those items are served. The dinner plate of 1950 measured ten inches across while today's plate is fully twelve inches, a two-inch increase that allows for the placement of 25 percent more food. Whatever the size and type of vessel we happen to be working with, we do endeavor to fill them. Once full, most of us accept it as our mission to ensure that nothing is left behind.

Chapter 2

Food Is Not the Enemy

I promise that it is not necessary to eat like a cave dweller, become a vegan (although restraining your saturated fat consumption is a worthy goal), limit yourself to cabbage soup or grapefruit, or cleanse your colon with coffee. Diets that have as their basis excessively restrictive nutritional practices or that encourage bizarre medical procedures as a means of weight loss should at the very least cause one to exercise careful consideration before enrolling. Weight loss is a process; it is not a science experiment. Are there foods that one would be wise to avoid? Absolutely. However, if eliminating those foods from your diet would make you miserable in the process, then ways must be found to include them, if perhaps only in a limited way.

Food selection is a very personal thing and is influenced by many factors, including cultural and religious preferences, upbringing, individual taste, availability and cost to name but a few. Whatever it is that motivates one to select a particular food item, the item itself has no evil intent. The most sinful appearing cupcake is after all inert, asking neither to be eaten nor ignored. Our antagonist is not food but rather how we respond to it. As cartoonist Walt Kelly observed, "We have met the enemy and he is us". We constantly sabotage our efforts to stay on the nutritional straight and narrow. Confronted with a choice between the aforementioned cupcake and a handful of carrot sticks, which would you choose? Dependent upon your mood and a host of other factors, you could decide either way. The enduring fact about diets is that each day presents new opportunities for successes and yes, failures. As is true with life itself, diets are a marathon not a sprint. It is important we look at the diet in its totality rather than how we performed on any single day. Let's not celebrate too loudly our short-term successes or bemoan our minor setbacks. No one who woke up overweight today was thin and fit yesterday. Just as weight gain occurs overtime, so too must weight loss.

Perhaps it is best we work to change our mindset relative to diet. To most people's way of thinking, the word diet refers to a process by which one's food intake is reduced in order to achieve weight loss. The alternative definition speaks in more general terms to the foods that an individual or an animal typically eats. For instance, it can be said an African elephant's diet consists of grasses, small plants, bushes, twigs, tree bark, roots, and fruit. Elephants and others that feed exclusively on plant materials are referred to as herbivores. On the other hand, those that eat principally meat are called carnivores. The human animal is neither one nor the other. We belong to a group referred to as omnivores. On this point, the rabid members of the vegan community and I differ. They would argue that humans are biologically adapted to eating plant materials; that, among other things, the shape of the human head is ill suited to dig into the carcasses of our prey. This is a lovely visual to be sure, but for me, aside from the point. I will not debate them on the taxonomy of our species, I will simply say that the vast majority of us can and do eat freely from both categories of food and thanks to the advent of meat departments, our head shape is not a limiting factor.

If you're one who chooses to have meat in your diet, fear not. Neither it nor the occasional doughnut spells ruin for your weight loss goals. We must account for the calories that come from those foods as with all foods we consume. Whatever their source, if you desire to lose weight then the calories you consume must be outstripped by the calories you burn. At the end of the day shedding pounds comes down to this very simple math equation: calories out must exceed calories in. Here too I am likely to get a great deal of push back from those who have made it their business to dispense nutrition information. Some among them might suggest that *when* you consume your calories is a factor or from what source your calories come. Still others would contend it is necessary to remove all processed foods from one's diet and eat only natural or organic foods. To them I would say, strictly as it relates to weight, these things don't matter.

Far be it from me to suggest that those who make diet more complex than it needs to be are motivated to do so. Only by making diet an otherwise unsolvable cryptogram can the experts compel the legions of the forlorn overweight to beat a path to their door or more correctly their website from which they can purchase a membership, DVDs, or other items, which will help them to achieve a lasting weight loss. To them I will be seen as a heretic. By espousing a philosophy, which is so at odds with theirs, how can they see me otherwise? I suppose they could argue that by writing this book I have thrown myself into the fray. Like the others, I could be said to have my own motivation, my own selfish personal interests. Sure, I'd like the book to be read but primarily because I believe it contains some basic truths.

Truths I expect many Americans, most especially those who do not have a weight problem, already hold true.

Diet is not a complex alchemy. People can eat the foods they enjoy with the understanding that the calories those foods represent must be paid for with activity. Therein lays the rub. The cost in activity of many of our more calorie-dense foods (the foods so many of us crave) is higher than most of us are willing to pay. Once that balance tilts in the direction of excess calories, even only slightly, weight gain occurs. A daily surplus of as little as 50 calories (the number of calories in a single Oreo cookie) would put us on a course to add more than five pounds in the span of one year.

This type of weight gain, frequently experienced in America, is what has been termed creeping obesity. It takes place slowly, incrementally. Changes like hair loss, the furrows in our brow or the so-called crow's feet are subtle and accrue overtime. When you look in a mirror, staring back at you is an image of yourself. You recognize the person as you, the changes that take place from one day to the next are not significant enough to be made note of, yet when multiplied by the number of days in a year or years in a decade those changes become more than noteworthy - they become alarming; so too, the changes in our weight.

Shall we simply resign ourselves to these changes or can they be averted? With respect to crow's feet and the like, I'm afraid that minus the use of Botox and/or cosmetic surgical procedures, it is an undeniable part of the aging process. We either accept it or do as actor John Derek (*Knock on Any Door*, 1949) suggested: "Live fast, die young and leave a good looking corpse". As an interesting and perturbing aside, I find it more than a little bit annoying that cosmetic companies cast teenage girls to model their age defying products as though the product and not the model's age is responsible for her youthful appeal.

In a similar way, those who hawk exercise equipment and diet programs use exceptionally fit individuals as examples of what you can achieve with one or both. They believe, and perhaps rightly so, that those of us who seek to improve our physical form will be influenced to choose their product(s) as a means to accomplish that purpose. Whether or not either would, what is undeniably true is that to drop pounds, we must both dial up our activity level and dial down our food intake. But to what extent one and the other? Surely, we cannot be asked to calculate the calories that are expended by each activity in which we engage. Neither should we be required to weigh, or in some other way measure, our foods in order to determine their caloric content. Our lives are full enough without enduring the added complication of such measures. However, without doing so, how can we be certain we're on a path to achieve our goals? The simple answer is to do less of one and more of the other.

Without counting our calories, we intuitively know that in order to lose weight we must begin by eating less. Without speaking about specific content, our meals must become proportionately smaller. Albert Einstein suggested that insanity be defined as doing the same thing repeatedly and expecting different results. If we accept that definition, it is insane for us to expect to lose weight by doing the same things that put us in the position where weight loss became necessary. Those who find themselves in this predicament must pause to reflect on the where, why, when, and what of their eating habits.

Here a critical self-examination is required. You must ask yourself, what are my triggers for eating? How can I modify my lifestyle to avoid those triggers? For some, rewiring the triggers will be difficult. As has been discussed, being overweight/obese is not an acute problem, but one that has developed during the course of many years; a product of an aberrant relationship with the food we eat, where food becomes something other than a fuel source. For whom among us is that not the case? Do any of us eat solely for the purpose of fueling our machines? We are by now many millennia removed from digging grubs out of the underbrush, and I for one am happy for it. Not intended solely as sustenance, but meant to satisfy, our food should not be merely life sustaining, it should also be life affirming. Just as intercourse is about more than procreation, so is eating about more than fuel. Though some may wish to do so, we cannot engage in sex whenever the mood strikes nor can we eat without restraint. Let's leave intemperate intercourse as a subject for another author and return to the aftermath of ill-restrained eating, it is after all that which has brought us this far.

There is nothing easy about weight loss. Even assuming you are able to identify the triggers to your overeating, modifying those behaviors will not come easily. It is not as if this revelation of overeating will hit you like an epiphany. I wouldn't expect to hear any overweight individuals announce with incredulity they had just come to the realization that they've been overeating all along. Overeating is the symptom, it is the why that needs to be addressed.

Let us assume for the sake of illustration that we identify watching television as one of our triggers. Some of us have developed the habit of mindlessly snacking while entranced by the soft glow of the television. On any given night, we can be seen consuming one chip or one cookie after another, oblivious to the affect that it will have on our waistline. When morning comes, we'll reflect upon our misdeed and it will occur to us anew that we lack the will to win this battle. Disheartened and dejected, we will confront the day certain in the knowledge that everyone we encounter is aware of our transgression and will judge us harshly for it.

Such are the travails of the overweight. To be the subject of another's scorn, real or imagined, is an especially burdensome cross to bear. If we carry this weight, we must cast it off if we are to achieve our goal. To the extent that we care about how others perceive us, we must first change how we perceive ourselves. Minus a change in self-perception, we will always be in our own mind incapable of succeeding or unworthy of success.

Let us now imagine ourselves free of self-doubt, convinced of the correctness of our journey, and committed to see it to its rightful conclusion. We must still deal with the anxiety that comes along with any major change in how we lead our lives. Divorce, the loss of a job, the death of a loved one, each of these events alters the course of our lives. Dependent upon the degree to which we find comfort in eating so too will a change in our eating habits. Though we often meet change with apprehension, the types of change about which we speak should instead be met with confidence. You are taking the first steps toward realizing a personal goal, toward taking control of your weight and everything tied to it.

If you haven't already done so, take time now to explore the root causes of your own issues with food. I don't intend to suggest that getting at these causes will be a simple matter. Nothing about the weight loss process is easy, but to be successful in the long term, you must begin by ferreting out the behaviors that brought you to this point. Armed with this information and the newfound confidence that comes from having fully committed to taking on this demon, it is now time to begin your journey.

Unlike others who offer advice on weight loss, I will not ask for early radical change in your food choices. What I propose is not dieting in the traditional sense, but rather altering the manner in which we go about our lives. Sure, for many that will involve changes to their diet, but more fundamentally, it will involve changes to their lifestyles, particularly as those changes affect weight. Getting back to the notion of calories in and calories out, it will be exceedingly difficult to accomplish your weight loss goals via changes in eating habits alone. Yet it is there where we begin. I will address the other half of that equation in subsequent chapters.

So, you say that rice cakes are not on your list of favorite foods, and neither kale nor bok choy is among your ten favorite vegetables. In fact, you couldn't name ten vegetables let alone have ten favorites. In this regard, you are not alone. The majority of Americans would not consider a rice cake to be an acceptable snack food, yet for that purpose it is ideally suited (except of course for those who hate them). As for vegetables, the variety of taste, color and texture they bring to our plates has all but been supplanted by the brown foods that have become the mainstay of the American diet. Since the early 1980s when the Reagan administration anointed pickle relish and ketchup as vegetables that which could be slathered on a bun became as close to a vegetable as many Americans dared to tread. If you are one such American, I will not (at least not yet) ask you to abandon your practices outright. Committing to this course was a courageous step, and although I want you to take each subsequent step confidently, I believe success will come from not asking for wholesale changes early. What I will ask is that you begin by ramping down the quantity of food you eat. In this case I am not asking you to weigh out your portions; I'm simply suggesting that your plate of today and going forward be less fully occupied. In addition, I want you to make an effort to leave some percentage of your meal on the plate when you leave the table (or wherever it is that you happen to be eating). Free yourself from the notion you must eat every morsel on your plate. In this instance, try to adopt the cat's mindset, which tells it that whatever it is eating now will not be its last.

Our tallest hurdles to surmount are those related to our perceptions and habits as they concern food. But surmount them we must. It may be that we won't glide over them, but we will ultimately put them behind us. To do so, I believe that our initial steps must be carefully trod. To ask too much at this early stage is to invite failure. Instead, the changes should be such that if we were to have someone else enact them on our behalf, we might not even be aware they were occurring. Nevertheless, in order to find a permanent place to roost in our eating strategies, the changes have to come about through conscious volition. We must choose to do this for ourselves, it cannot be chosen for us. While we may accept direction even in so accepting, we are choosing.

A final choice I ask you to consider now is to limit your calories consumed in the form of beverages. Because beverages contribute little to the sense of satiety or fullness, while at the same time providing a disproportionately high calorie load, they are particularly problematic for those whose desire it is to lose weight. Compounding their limitations, many beverages offer little nutrition. The best among them provide nothing you cannot find in solid food while the worst deliver only slightly more than flavored sugar water. Even America's morning obsession coffee, has become a bad actor. During the days of my youth, coffee was little more than a caffeine delivery system. Black, it contributed few calories to our daily intake. Fast forward to the present day and the coffee served up to us by the local barista in some cases bears little resemblance to that which percolated on our kitchen counters not so many years ago. Today's brews are not only significantly larger, they are also augmented and embellished through the addition of various types of syrups and powders that, while they no doubt alter the taste, also alter the fat and calorie count so much that some of the selections push up to and beyond five hundred calories. Few among us can tolerate a calorie hit of that magnitude and not be affected. Therefore, if your engine requires an a.m. caffeine kick-start, then have your coffee, but please leave its accouterments for those in line behind you.

Nutritional Information for Popular Coffee Based Beverages				
	Size (oz)	Calories	Saturated Fat (grams)	Sugars (grams)
Starbucks Coffee Company				
Caffe Latte	16	190	4.5	17
Caffe Mocha	16	330	9	35
Cappuccino	16	120	2	-
Caramel Macchiato	16	240	3.5	32
Cinnamon Dolce Latte	16	330	8	40
Chocolate Cookie Crumble Frappuccino	16	460	13	60
Caramel Ribbon Crunch Frappuccino	16	560	12	93
Peet's Coffee				
Caffe Latte	16	260	8	20
Caffe Mocha	16	330	8	35
Vanilla Caffe Latte	16	340	8	43
Chai Freddo	16	350	4	62
Caramel Caffe Freddo	16	370	3	68
Dark Chocolate Caramel Freddo	16	420	4	76

Dunkin' Donuts				
Dunkaccino	14	350	13	38
Iced Mocha Swil Latte	16	350	6	51
Caramel Coffee Coolata	16	390	6	72
Mocha Coffe Coolata	16	800	25	96
Caribou Coffee				
Latte	18	200	5	19
Chai Tea Latte	18	330	5	50
Caramel High Rise	18	360	11.5	40
Turtle Mocha	18	580	20	65

Table assembled using information collected from
the respective coffeehouse's websites

Chapter 3

The Dreaded Calorie and What It Means To You

Each of the foods we consume, as well as many of the beverages we drink, carries with it a specific calorie count. For the purposes of this discussion, think of calories as the fuel that powers our engines. Minus this fuel, we would all stall alongside the roads of our lives, incapable of executing the simplest of tasks. For the vast majority of Americans, it is not the absence of fuel that concerns us but rather the over abundance of it.

Unlike our cars, trucks, buses, planes et al., the human body has no finite fuel storage reservoirs. When filling your car's tank, it is only possible to add as much gasoline as it will bear. If you continue to fill beyond the tank's capacity, the portion that exceeds the capacity spills out onto the ground. For better or worse, we humans have tanks that can adjust for the amount of fuel onboard. Although not often appreciated as such, this is a highly evolved system. Intended to provide for us during times of deprivation, our fuel reserves (alternatively known as fat) are now seldom utilized. They are instead progressively added to seeking ever-higher levels until some unimagined cataclysm befalls us or until we decide to act.

Barring cataclysm, we must assert our will. But what is the nature of the task? If it is fuel that we are storing then it must be fuel that we expend in order to lighten our load. Would that it were as easy to peel off as it was to apply. While weight comes off in the same way it was added, which is to say calorie by calorie, it is a challenge to burn through that which is stored. Complicating matters, we always seem to be in a hurry to rid ourselves of it. We spend our time adding and then rush to subtract, usually motivated by some upcoming social event. Whether it is swimsuit season, a wedding, or a class reunion, we scramble to look our best by setting what in many cases are completely unrealistic weight loss goals. A quick search of the Internet reveals multiple sites that offer nonsurgical weight loss solutions that promise to take off twenty pounds or more in thirty days time. Short of lopping off a limb and having that add to the total such claims are flights of fancy, appealing notions but not much more particularly given what is known about true weight loss.

Still, one nationally advertised supplement offers a rapid solution to weight loss woes. The plan calls for you to supplant your daily food intake with a powdered drink mix, that's right - eat nothing! Three times per day for the first week, you add the powder to some water, drink it down, and give your muscles of mastication some well deserved time off. Assuming you survive the first week, weeks two and beyond allow for the introduction of a small salad at lunch with the continued use of the supplement at breakfast and dinner. At approximately 180 calories per serving, using this product will, of course, yield weight loss, but at what cost? This weight loss solution does nothing more than reinforce the binge-starve eating behaviors that are characteristic of serial dieters. As such, it and programs like it should not be thought of as reasonable or healthy options when one is considering weight loss strategies. In contradistinction to programs such as that outlined above, I favor a more rational and sensible approach that aims to alter how we relate to food.

Understanding the simple mathematics of weight loss is part of the process that leads to a more wholesome relationship with the food we eat. In order to arrive at that place, let's look at the numbers that underlie weight loss.

Accepting some difference of opinion on the actual number, a pound of fat is roughly equivalent to thirty-five hundred calories. Using that as our number, we must subtract some portion of that number from our daily caloric intake (assuming we are to accomplish our purpose through diet alone) in order to achieve weight loss. Mind you, we will be subtracting the portion not necessarily from what you have been eating, but rather what you should be eating. To pick a number, let's say that your age, gender, body type and activity level allow you to eat twenty-two hundred calories a day to stay at your present weight. Those twenty-two hundred calories are in effect allocated to us to meet our daily energy needs. Continuing with this example 60 percent of the total comes from what is referred to as basal metabolism, or the energy cost associated with keeping the body functioning while at rest. An additional 10 percent is designated for the energy demands tied to the digesting and processing of the food we eat. Yes, we're even burning calories while we ingest them. These two numbers are effectively fixed, which is to say that they are not within our ability to regulate. The number we do have control over are the calories burned through physical activity. Accounting for approximately 30 percent of our daily total this number is the key variable in our quest to lose weight. This is the number that allows us to increase the calorie cost of living our lives.

However, even through its manipulation, reaching the aforementioned unrealistic weight loss goal of twenty pounds in thirty days would require we eat nothing during those thirty days and even then, we would come up short. More realistic would be the idea of losing a pound per week. Even at that, you would be required to reduce your caloric intake by more than 20 percent per day down to approximately seventeen hundred calories. In this example, it is easy to see the affect that a five hundred-calorie coffee drink might have on your efforts to peel off the pounds. Here again I reiterate, it is not an easy process yet still ultimately doable given a rock-solid sense of self-confidence and determination.

Other digits we need to consider are the numbers four, four and nine. These are the ballpark numbers of calories found in one gram of carbohydrate, protein, and fat respectively. They are important numbers because they provide strong testimony for the caution we must exercise when eating fatty foods in particular. As the numbers indicate, fat contains more than twice the calories found in either carbohydrate or protein.

Pause for a moment to consider the ramifications. By unit volume, you can eat two times as much carbohydrate or protein as fat for a similar calorie cost. What this means in practical terms is that you can eat twice as much broccoli as ice cream, eat twice as many asparagus spears (sorry, no butter) as cheesecake, or twice the number of black bean burgers as rashes of bacon. This leads many to wonder, why is it that everything that tastes good is bad for you? I will not at this time discuss which foods are good for us and which are bad. It is our mission to exercise control over your calorie consumption. If your present diet is over-weighted on the side of fatty foods, that process becomes more vexing. Remembering that at present we hope to accomplish a reduction in the number of calories consumed without instituting a radical change in what you eat, opting for less of the foods you enjoy rather than more of the foods you do not enjoy. However, if your preferred meal consists of a hamburger, fries and a shake, one such meal could break your calorie bank for the entire day. Even if you were able to limit yourself to one such meal per day, would such a scheme be advisable?

I will answer this question by way of analogy. Think of your body as a fire burning on a cold winter's night. That fire warms your home most efficiently if it burns at a steady state. Rather than stoke the fire to burn intensely then smolder out, it is preferable for the sake of consistent heat to manage your fire to burn evenly. We can say the same of our bodies. It is more desirable to provide your body with measured amounts of fuel (calories) throughout the day than to offer it a single massive meal at any one point.

Nutritional Information for Popular Fast Food Meals					
	Calories	Saturated Fat (grams)		Calories	Saturated Fat (grams)
Arby's			**Burger King**		
Angus Three Cheese Bacon Burger	630	11	Double Whopper	830	17
Large Curly Fries	630	5	Large Fries	500	3.5
Large Chocolate Shake	570	10	Large Chocolate Shake	980	17
TOTAL	1930	26	TOTAL	2310	37.5
Carl's Jr.			**Dairy Queen**		
Super Bacon $6 Cheeseburger	1040	26	Flamethrower Grill Burger	740	16
Large Natural Cut Fries	460	22	Large Fries	490	3.5
Large Chocolate Shake	690	24	Large Chocolate Shake	940	20
TOTAL	2190	72	TOTAL	2170	39.5
In & Out Burger			**Jack In The Box**		
Double Double	670	18	Bacon Ultimate Cheeseburger	906	24
Large Fries	395	5	Large Fries	557	2
Large Chocolate Shake	590	19	Large Chocolate Shake	798	26
TOTAL	1655	42	TOTAL	2261	52
Johnny Rockets			**McDonald's**		
Bacon Cheddar Double	1770	50	Double Quarter Pounder with Cheese	750	19
Large Fries	480	3	Large Fries	500	12
Oreo Cookies & Cream Shake	1030	33	Large Chocolate Shake	700	12
TOTAL	3280	86	TOTAL	1950	43

Sonic			Wendy's		
SuperSonic Bacon Double Cheeseburger	1240	35	Baconator	980	27
Large Fries	470	4	Large Fries	500	4.5
Large Chocolate Shake	1410	41	Large Chocolate Frosty	880	11
TOTAL	3120	80	TOTAL	2360	42.5

Table assembled using information collected from the respective restaurant's websites

Short of the "one meal a day" diet plan (after all we are not goldfish), how can you find room in your diet for a burger and fries? I see two options. The first is to pare down the size of each serving stopping just short of the "homeopathic burger," which is diluted to the point where it only contains the essence of the burger and none of its calories (an admittedly weak attempt to take the edge off what is for many the very serious subject of weight loss), or increase the calories one expends during the course of the day. While I continue to advocate for calorie reduction through diet modification, it is important to consider the role that exercise (here I use the term broadly to include all activities that increase the calorie cost of living our lives) plays in the management of our weight.

Chapter 4

Choose to Move

Where weight loss is concerned, exercise and calorie restriction are two sides of the same coin. It would be difficult to achieve sustained weight loss without combining elements of both. Up to this point, we have discussed implementing a program whereby we look to shed pounds through diet manipulation alone. As the numbers indicated, such a program is at best a tough row to hoe. The long and laborious task of dropping a few pounds a month has potential of leaving some dieters demoralized, and why not? Given what for many must be perceived as a huge personal sacrifice in the form of restricted food intake, one would hope to realize results that are more significant. Adding exercise to the process would certainly aid in that cause.

Exercise is the only legitimate way in which you can, in effect, up the ante by increasing the number of calories you expend.

For those whose weight remains constant, there is an equilibrium maintained between the calories consumed and the calories expended. In order to lose weight, we must offset that equilibrium by pushing it in the direction of calorie deficit. We have begun to do so by limiting our intake, but in order to make the deficit steeper still, we must ratchet up activity. I admit that life, as it is presently lead with its many conveniences, makes it possible for a large number of us to avoid unnecessary toil.

Doubtlessly, these conveniences have contributed to our increased girth. It is no mystery that when we eat more and do less, we gain weight. We are not the only species in the animal kingdom who suffer this fate. Those animals that spend their lives as zoo attractions are not made to work for their food as are their counterparts in the wild. These under-exercised and potentially overfed animals are no less susceptible to weight increases and the diseases associated therewith. Perhaps, unlike those animals, we have the ability to renounce our conveniences. We are not duty bound to utilize escalators, elevators and other automated people movers. In fact, I believe rejecting such devices is a critical first step toward increasing the energy demand we place upon our bodies.

It is not necessary for us to be ultramarathoners; we do not need to be professional athletes, in truth, we don't need to be athletes at all. What we can't be are layabouts, loafers, couch potatoes. Instead of seeking shortcuts toward the completion of a particular task, why not consider options that would make the job physically more demanding. Rather than blow your leaves, why not rake them. Instead of hosing down your walk, choose a broom. In lieu of paying your neighbor's son to mow the lawn, mow it yourself. If the market is around the corner, and the bank is down the block, instead of burning the fuel in your car, how about burning some of your own? Or, what about this, rather than waiting for the parking stall nearest the store to become available, why not park in the one farthest away? If you've never noticed before, that parking space is the one you'll rarely find occupied.

These suggestions don't amount to exercise in the way we have come to think of it. You won't need your running shoes or have to drive to the gym; these exercises are right outside your front door. They may be small things when you look at them individually, but they are significant when part of a larger whole

I realize that the thought of purposefully attempting to increase your workload is counterintuitive. But if life asks less of us, then we must finds ways to ask more of ourselves. Just as we have to decide to make a downward adjustment in what we eat so too must we decide to make an upward adjustment in our activity level. It is both as simple and as complicated as that: simple in the thought of it, complicated in its execution.

Oftentimes when presented with such a quandary, we turn to the experts for their take on how to proceed. Because we have neither the time nor the expertise to critically evaluate the relevant research, we rely upon them to do that for us, to analyze the data and disseminate it in a way that will be most easily understood. The problem is that too many of these experts have their own ax to grind, their own wares to pedal. When such is the case, personal bias may enter into the equation and muddy up the interpretation of the data and the message that grows out of that interpretation.

As it relates to research in the area of nutrition, when multiple experts arrive at differing opinions, confusion ensues. What do we do when confronted with conflicting opinion? Either we choose the expert whose credentials we hold in highest esteem, or we select the opinion more consistent with our own. In either case, the role of the expert is greatly diminished. When it comes to medical matters, nutrition included, we want answers not conjecture, not speculation, and certainly not a sales pitch.

While opinions relative to the need for exercise as a means of mediating weight loss may differ, the differences have more to do with how much or in what form, rather than whether it needs to be done at all. I suspect people would find themselves on a philosophical island were they to advocate against the inclusion of exercise in any well-designed weight loss program. Far from advocating against it, I am a strong proponent of exercise in general and as a facilitator for weight loss. However, as was the case for my recommendations relative to diet, one's initial foray into exercise should not overreach. The goal here is not to bring about drastic change but rather achievable and sustainable change.

If you are not a natural exerciser, one who has an affinity for it, it is unreasonable to expect that you will simply adopt exercise in place of your previously more sedentary lifestyle. As the saying goes, you cannot make a silk purse out of a sow's ear, but I do think that it is possible to make an exerciser out of someone who had no prior interest in being seen as such. In my estimation, the key to a successful transformation lies in proceeding with measured steps. The failure to appreciate the importance of these steps has lead some to create boot camp style exercise programs while others have developed commercial home exercise regimens for the mass-market. For the experienced exerciser, such programs can be useful tools in their quest to achieve greater levels of fitness. However, for the first time, or novice exerciser. these programs may be a bridge too far. This is especially true for those who are significantly overweight. Imposing high-intensity exercise on such a person can reinforce their preexisting negative association with exercise in general, and worse, may yield undesirable medical consequences. In a very real way dieters must learn to walk before they can run.

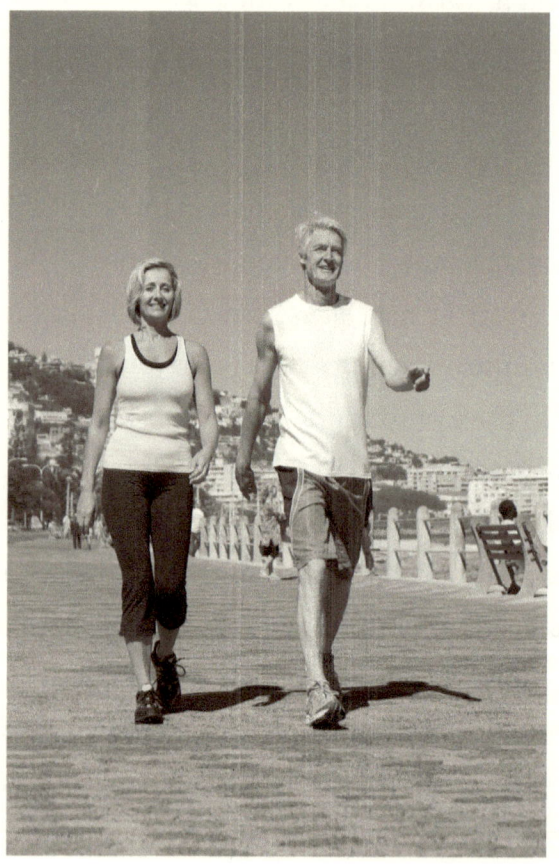

At the age of sixty-four, Diana Nyad swam the 110 miles from Cuba to the Florida Keys in fifty-three hours. Her mantra for the challenge was to "find a way". In walking, you will not face a challenge nearly so arduous, but in its execution you, like Nyad, must "find a way".

Walking is underappreciated as an exercise modality. Too many imagine or have been made to believe that exercise must be vigorous in order to be beneficial. For those not favorably disposed to exercise of that description, walking is an excellent alternative. Because it requires no special equipment or specific facility, one can walk virtually anywhere. Neither does it require a particular time commitment. Wherever or whenever the opportunity presents, walk.

In a perfect world, you would be able to do so continuously for thirty minutes or more; however, if your schedule does not allow or you are otherwise unable, it is possible to carve that time up into smaller segments, perhaps multiple fifteen-minute bouts as opposed to one mega walk. Whatever the case may be, if vigorous exercise is not to your liking, let walking form the foundation of your exercise program. If even that strikes you as repugnant, find a friend with whom you can walk, or try listening to an audio book, or use the walk as an opportunity to catch up with friends and family members via a cell phone. Sure, the calories you expend while doing so will not equal those burned during intense exercise of a similar duration, but that is not the point. Remember our objective is to increase the calorie cost as we navigate through our lives. Success at this level invites opportunities to increase our exercise load down the road.

Calories Burned While Walking (One Mile)

Weight: 110 lbs.			Weight: 120 lbs.			Weight: 130 lbs.			Weight: 140 lbs.		
Speed (mph)	Time (mins.)	Calories Burned	Speed (mph)	Time (mins.)	Calories Burned	Speed (mph)	Time (mins.)	Calories Burned	Speed (mph)	Time (mins.)	Calories Burned
2.0	30	62	2.0	30	68	2.0	30	74	2.0	30	80
2.5	24	60	2.5	24	65	2.5	24	71	2.5	24	76
3.0	20	55	3.0	20	60	3.0	20	65	3.0	20	70
3.5	17	54	3.5	17	59	3.5	17	63	3.5	17	68
4.0	15	62	4.0	15	68	4.0	15	74	4.0	15	79
4.5	13	79	4.5	13	86	4.5	13	93	4.5	13	100
5.0	12	80	5.0	12	87	5.0	12	94	5.0	12	102

Weight: 150 lbs.			Weight: 160 lbs.			Weight: 170 lbs.			Weight: 180 lbs.		
Speed (mph)	Time (mins.)	Calories Burned	Speed (mph)	Time (mins.)	Calories Burned	Speed (mph)	Time (mins.)	Calories Burned	Speed (mph)	Time (mins.)	Calories Burned
2.0	30	85	2.0	30	91	2.0	30	96	2.0	30	102
2.5	24	82	2.5	24	87	2.5	24	93	2.5	24	98
3.0	20	75	3.0	20	80	3.0	20	85	3.0	20	90
3.5	17	73	3.5	17	78	3.5	17	83	3.5	17	88
4.0	15	85	4.0	15	91	4.0	15	96	4.0	15	102
4.5	13	107	4.5	13	114	4.5	13	121	4.5	13	129
5.0	12	109	5.0	12	116	5.0	12	123	5.0	12	131

Weight: 190 lbs.			Weight: 200 lbs.			Weight: 210 lbs.			Weight: 220 lbs.		
Speed (mph)	Time (mins.)	Calories Burned	Speed (mph)	Time (mins.)	Calories Burned	Speed (mph)	Time (mins.)	Calories Burned	Speed (mph)	Time (mins.)	Calories Burned
2.0	30	108	2.0	30	114	2.0	30	119	2.0	30	125
2.5	24	103	2.5	24	109	2.5	24	114	2.5	24	120
3.0	20	95	3.0	20	100	3.0	20	105	3.0	20	110
3.5	17	93	3.5	17	98	3.5	17	103	3.5	17	107
4.0	15	108	4.0	15	113	4.0	15	119	4.0	15	125
4.5	13	136	4.5	13	143	4.5	13	150	4.5	13	157
5.0	12	138	5.0	12	145	5.0	12	152	5.0	12	160

Weight: 250 lbs.			Weight: 275 lbs.			Weight: 300 lbs.					
Speed (mph)	Time (mins.)	Calories Burned	Speed (mph)	Time (mins.)	Calories Burned	Speed (mph)	Time (mins.)	Calories Burned			
2.0	30	142	2.0	30	156	2.0	30	170			
2.5	24	136	2.5	24	150	2.5	24	164			
3.0	20	133	3.0	20	146	3.0	20	159			
3.5	17	130	3.5	17	143	3.5	17	156			
4.0	15	142	4.0	15	156	4.0	15	170			
4.5	13	159	4.5	13	175	4.5	13	191			
5.0	12	182	5.0	12	200	5.0	12	218			

In a consistent and constructive fashion, what we are actually attempting to accomplish is a reworking of attitudes toward both food and exercise. As it pertains to the latter, we want to bring you to a place where you cannot only accept it, but also embrace it as an important component of your daily regimen. We look to rejigger your past perceptions about exercise as an onerous and unpleasant process and instead, instill the thought that it can be enjoyable and ultimately rewarding. I do not believe we can bring you to that mindset by clubbing you over the head. Others metaphorically do just that (see *Biggest Losers*). They seem to use exercise as a form of punishment for dietary misdeeds. We will help you to lose the weight, they seem to say, but to do so, you must perform a punitive series of exercises. I have to wonder what it is that motivates such practices.

I prefer to believe the people behind these strategies have as their sincere intent the desire to assist others to achieve their weight loss goals. However, the jaded, cynical side of me questions whether it doesn't have more to do with TV ratings and time constraints imposed by a TV season. To draw in an audience, programs of that ilk must maximize the drama, and as it pertains to weight loss, drama comes in the form of rapid reduction and the battle to bring it about. Sadly many of those who attain the reductions are unable to retain them. Those who guided them to the losses failed to inculcate the attitudes, habits, and behaviors that would make it possible to maintain or build upon the weight loss. Consequently, a significant number of those tortured souls fell back into prior patterns and became what I refer to as nutritional recidivists. Quickly abandoning the unsustainable exercise and dietary practices, they regained the weight not long ago lost.

Those around them may perceive the return of the weight as an indication of personal weakness or as a kind of character flaw. They may ask, how could he/she allow him/herself to regain all of the weight they had lost? If this question were asked of me, I might say that while they ultimately bear the responsibility, perhaps they did not have the tools necessary to succeed long-term. The tools to which I refer are those that allow dieters to make the correct decisions when confronted with nutritional and exercise choices. To discern which choices will keep dieters moving forward and which might prevent them from doing so. It is neither possible nor desirable for dieters to have their every move monitored. The programs most likely to engender success are those that provide their subscribers with the knowledge and skills needed to make determinations independently.

For those free from the constraints of being overweight, the idea that such skills are needed might seem absurd on the face of it. Such a person might contend that the options are really quite simple, particularly as it relates to exercise.

As Yoda said to Luke Skywalker, "Do or do not, there is no try". However, for those who have spent their lives overweight, the idea of doing exercise, whatever the form, is fraught with perils of its own. The weight that they carry with them is not strictly physical. An emotional weight is an even greater impediment to exercise. To those who carry this weight, be mindful of the limitations it imposes. Do not allow your progress to be encumbered by the thoughts you may have about how others perceive your efforts to engage in exercise. Most who witness your exertions would celebrate them with you, for those who would not, let them be damned.

The act of losing weight is a singularly selfish one. Sure, spouses and children will benefit, but it must be principally for yourself that you do this. If it is through the exhortations of others that you have embarked on this journey, your chances of success diminish. Take this on for your own well-being. Accept the support of those who offer it and reject the comments of the disbelievers and naysayers, and let exercise be the instrument that helps you to make the most of the body you inhabit.

In a national advertising campaign, one large pharmaceutical company employs a variation of Isaac Newton's First Law of Motion to promote an anti-inflammatory drug. The company uses the tagline, "A body in motion tends to stay in motion". Newton's law states that whether a body is at rest or in motion, it will continue in that state unless acted upon by an external force. Rest will always have its place, but with it comes an inclination toward inactivity, a resistance to movement. To achieve your goals, exercise, activity, movement, and motion must find their way into your daily routine. As the law applies to this book, *you* must become the force that gives motion to your body.

Chapter 5

When the Cheering Fades

I have spent most of my career providing care for and counsel to elite-level athletes. During the course of my nearly thirty years of doing so, I have borne witness to some surprisingly poor eating habits. I suspect many recreational athletes and/or aspiring professional athletes imagine that the difference between them and those who have risen to the highest levels of sports comes down to nutrition. If they were to learn and apply the secrets of sports nutrition, they too could earn handsome livings chasing, kicking, throwing, hitting, catching, or shooting a ball. The reality as I have come to know it is that while nutrition is a factor, it is not *the* factor. The simple truth is that professional athletes are for the most part young people who eat as young people eat, which is to say without regard to consequences. And for the professional athlete, the consequences are few. Such is the wonder of being an athlete. The physical demands of their occupations allow for increased calorie consumption to offset those expended during practice and play. For many athletes, this becomes what is in effect a nutritional free pass. Eat whatever you choose because as an athlete, you have uncommon wiggle room where calories are concerned.

Among athletes competing in the most physically demanding sports tolerances of four- to five thousand calories and more per day are common. When preparing for the 2012 Olympic Games in London, American swimmer Ryan Lochte famously consumed ten thousand calories per day. Whether true or not I cannot say. These mythic stories tend to have only the loosest connections to reality, but it is a challenge that too many Americans would like to take on. The problem is, only the smallest percentages of us burn calories at a rate close to that number, for the rest of us, it amounts to additional pounds put on in a hurry. Even for athletes, those who could sustain an intake beyond five thousand calories would be few and far between. For those who can, it becomes a bit of a double-edged sword in that they can be significantly less discriminate in the quantity and quality of food they eat, but ultimately this too will end. Because the athlete's career is a relatively short one, that end comes before many are prepared to accept it, at least in terms of what it means for his or her nutritional practices.

Although many athletes retire at a relatively early age, the end of their playing careers signals what for many is a steep decline in activity. Suddenly, they are no longer performing the activities that had given them so much latitude in their food choices. Gone are the weeks during which they would spend twelve or more hours working out. In their place are workout schedules more akin to that of most other Americans, something approaching ninety minutes per week. Perhaps it is retirement alone, or retirement combined with the lingering effects of musculoskeletal injury, but either way, the calories burned drop off sharply, and unless adjustments are made on the intake side, weight gain follows.

Disciplined though they may have been in their workout regimes, few athletes were similarly well disciplined in their eating habits. Although their professional careers may be short, most athletes participate in their sport of choice for many years before they are able to translate it into a paycheck. It is during their formative years - first as recreational, and then high school and then college athletes - that poor nutritional practices take seed. While each has sat through lectures extolling the virtues of proper food choice vis a vis sports performance, most athletes continue to dance with the foods that brought them to the professional ranks. Lest you be led astray by athlete interviews to the contrary, pizza, ice cream, candy, and the like are no less prominently featured in their diets than in that of most Americans.

Painting with the same broad brush used in the previous paragraph, it has been my experience that athletes are less averse to eating fruits and vegetables than are many Americans. According to the Centers for Disease Control, only about 25 percent of American adults eat the recommended five servings per day of fruits and vegetables, while less than 25 percent of adolescents do likewise. This could be seen as a silver lining for the otherwise dark cloud that portends trouble ahead, in the form of weight gain, for the retired athlete.

While making a modest downward adjustment in calories consumed has been a guiding principle in the text to this point, such an adjustment may not be enough to stave off weight gain for the retired athlete. For those whose activity levels fall off precipitously, there must be a concomitant decrease in the quantity of food consumed, or more correctly, the calories taken in by each food eaten. Bearing in mind that during their careers, athletes may ingest up to and in some cases beyond five thousand calories per day, shaving off five hundred calories here or there will likely be insufficient if the goal is to remain at their playing weight. For this reason, playing weight quickly becomes a distant memory. The list of former players who have made significant additions to their physical forms is long and illustrious. It includes past Heisman Trophy winners, Super Bowl MVPs, Hall of Famers, Cy Young Award winners, rookies of the year, Stanley Cup champions, in short, all who have donned a uniform will become susceptible to an expanding waistline, and in this regard they are no different from us. Among those whose sport allowed for them to participate while fat the forecast is even grimmer. I do not know whom it was that suggested inside every fat athlete is an even fatter one trying to get out, but it is certainly supported by the evidence.

In an interview posted on CNN *Living* (January 2013), former tennis superstar turned author, Martina Navratilova offers advice to those who, like her, have retired from sport. Her recommendation, "Find another sport that you can really improve at, that you can get excited about, and have fun". Solid advice, Martina! I echo her sentiments and encourage not only former athletes but everyone to find a sport or activity about which they can become passionate.

A popular choice among retired athletes is golf. I suppose on some level it fills a need to be competitive, and if that is what motivates you to participate then by all means be competitive. Insofar as where it ranks among calorie burning activities, I think Mark Twain best summarized it when he said, "Golf is a good walk spoiled". At the time he made the comment, Twain was referring to the frustrations attendant to conveying that small-dimpled ball from the tee to the cup.

Today, with those frustrations still in place, the advent of golf carts has done more to spoil the walk. From an exercise perspective, the walk is most fruitful. Interspersed with efforts to club the ball around the course, the walk is that aspect of the game that yields the highest number of calories burned. In this one respect, I think being a bad golfer has its advantages since it is for such a golfer that the path to the hole is seldom a straight line. Regardless your skill level, if you're holding golf out as an exercise activity then you must leave the cart in the barn.

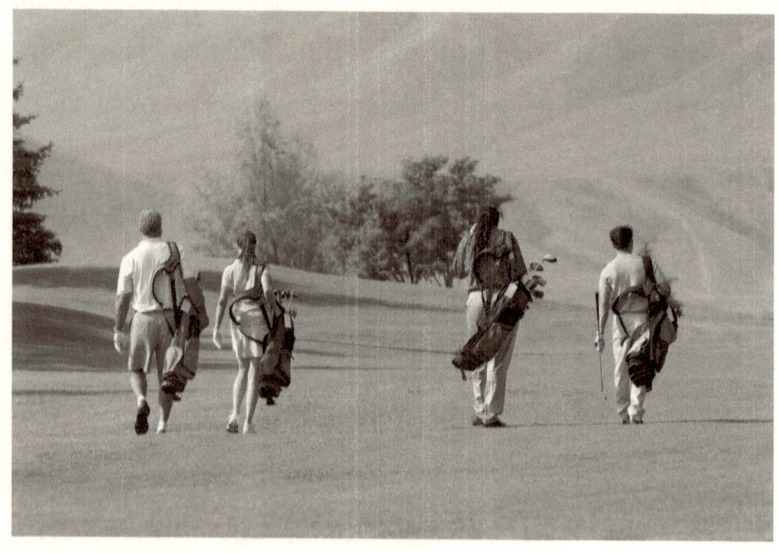

If you're a golfer, embrace that aspect of the game that yields the greatest return in terms of calories burned – walk the course.

Whether a former athlete or not, leaving the cart in favor of walking causes us to rethink the role that convenience plays in our lives. Devices intended to save us effort and time literally surround us. But what becomes of the time and effort we save? If those conveniences buy us time to perform other meaningful tasks, we are better for them. If, on the other hand, they simply afford us more idle time, we have gained nothing. We were never intended to be a sedentary species; such a lifestyle runs counter to our bodies' chemistry. To function at our optimum we must achieve a balance between our energy intake and expenditure. To the extent the labor saved by our conveniences upsets that balance, efforts must be made to find alternatives. Ours may not be the largest brain in the animal kingdom, but it is certainly the most nimble. We inherently know what we must do; the problem lies in the doing.

Chapter 6

The Truth Shall Set You Free

In the darkness that is ignorance, fraud and misinformation flourish. Within this context, the ignorance I refer to is not equivalent to stupidity, but is a product of a lack of familiarity or experience with a particular subject. Because even the brightest among us cannot be knowledgeable on all subjects, it is at times necessary to seek opinions from those more informed than we. For better or worse, this is how we learn about the outside world.

For those aged forty and older, think about those questions you asked of your parents and teachers; questions that if asked of your father in particular, were often answered with, "Ask your mother". Many of life's greatest conundrums were left unanswered by the sources we depended upon.

Fortunately, in the fullness of time, we discovered the answers for ourselves - girls don't have cooties and the moon is not made of swiss cheese. Today, whatever our age, whatever our question, the answer is but a few keystrokes away. However, like our questions of old, the answers are only as good as the veracity of the source providing them.

With regard to matters of fact, a single unassailable correct answer would be the only appropriate response. If asked who was the sixteenth President of the United States, the answer will always be Abraham Lincoln. There can be no correct alternative response. We cannot say the same of questions for which no single true answer is known. In such cases, the answers proffered will always involve some amount of theorizing, hypothesizing, and, yes, a measure of guessing, regardless how emphatically stated. It is important, therefore, that we become proficient at separating fact from opinion. Again referencing Lincoln, it is a fact he was shot while attending a play at Ford's Theatre on April 14th, 1865. The thought that he was our most beloved president would be a matter of opinion and hotly debated by those from the South in the latter half of the nineteenth century.

How, you must be asking yourself, does any of this relate to medical matters in general or dieting in particular? The short answer is that much about medicine, up to and including the supplementary discipline of nutrition, involves guessing - educated guessing - but guessing nevertheless.

Doubtlessly, those who are in the business of administering to the human machine would not warmly receive such a claim. To those who do, I will not suggest that progress has not been made, yet it remains my belief that what is definitively known about the human body could be written longhand on the head of a pin. Here I admit to a bit of hyperbole, but it goes to make the point that we are nowhere near to understanding the riddle that is the human organism. On those issues where certainty does not exist, opinion exists in profusion. There is no better example of this than in the area of weight management.

Thus far, I have promoted my view that weight gain is a product of increased consumption and decreased exertion. This is the truth as I know the truth to be. Surely, others will challenge some of my thoughts, if not my central thesis, and earn a measure of public support for doing so, after all, the notion of self-determination as it applies to weight is certain to have its detractors.

In a world where the most famous among us fail to accept responsibility for their actions, why should the rest of us take responsibility for ours? Lance Armstrong counter-accused, Pete Rose covered-up, Alex Rodriguez cast a smoke screen, Bernie Madoff deceived, Bill Clinton obfuscated, John Edwards falsified and the appropriately named Anthony Weiner denied. Add in former National League Most Valuable Player, Ryan Braun, and erstwhile South

Carolina Governor Mark Sanford, a man who famously claimed to be hiking the Appalachian Trail while he was in fact sleeping with his mistress in Argentina, and you have a small but illustrious sampling of those who chose to prevaricate rather than own up to their transgressions. This rogue's gallery of false witnesses has, each during their own time, caused us to scratch our heads in utter amazement at the lengths some will go to conceal their misdeeds. The lessons that have grown out of their ultimate exposure seem quickly forgotten, as many more have lied, and many more *will* in order to protect their place in society. Given the role that these people and those like them play in forming policy, is it any wonder that it is our inclination to look outside ourselves when ascribing blame?

If being overweight is your problem, please know it is not my purpose to blame you. It is my purpose to help you to understand the issues underlying the problem. Where causation is concerned, which is the more likely explanation? A) Your weight gain is hormonal, or tied to an undiagnosed kidney or liver problem, or it has its origin in a food sensitivity; or B) It is the result of an energy imbalance where too much is coming in and not enough is going out. Here, the adage commonly called upon by medical professionals seems appropriate, "When you hear hoofbeats don't think zebras". Physicians who employ this adage are typically attempting to illustrate, through the use of metaphor, that the most likely explanation for an illness or ailment is probably the correct one. That said it will require only a small investment of time to find some number of folks who imagine that their cough is not the result of the common cold, but rather a symptom of an especially virulent strain of tuberculosis.

I do not know what it says about us that on those occasions when we become patients we tend to magnify our complaints and imagine that our condition is much worse than others believe it to be. Yet we do, and finding people to support us in our delusion is often a simple matter so long as we pay them for that support. Enter "weight management" into your search engine of choice, and you will discover millions willing to provide that support. And why not when the US weight loss industry racks up an estimated sixty billion dollars in annual sales? In order to take their slice of the pie, some practitioners will happily sell you their pill, potion, poultice, or program all carefully marketed to ensnare you in what is often the false promise of rapid weight loss. For those who have become so ensnared, let that deception be the last. Others will surely work to tempt you with the next best thing, but resist their promise. Put their advertising to the test. Are they presenting facts or opinion dressed up as the same? In the world of commercial weight loss, the distinction may not be obvious. They may begin with a fact then twist and distort it until the truth has been wrung out of it.

Like snake oil of old, today's elixirs are sold with little fear of repercussions. Because the prevailing laws that regulate the manufacture and distribution of these products do not require prior FDA (Food and Drug Administration) approval, companies operate with near impunity. Their charge is to ensure the products they produce are safe and their marketing claims are truthful. When you leave a fox to oversee your hen house, don't expect to find your chickens warm and cozy when you return. Still, there must be some consequence for brazenly deceiving the consumer. Again, borrowing from the wit of Twain, "It ain't what you don't know that gets you into trouble. It's what you know for sure that just ain't so" [sic]. If you claim your product accomplishes a particular purpose and repeatedly fails to do so, surely then the FDA would act. The truth is only under the most egregious of circumstances will the FDA be compelled to intervene. By that time, the company will be flush with cash and those who purchased their product will be, in all likelihood, no closer to their goal of significant weight loss.

However rare recalls might be, they do occur. In an article published in JAMA (*Journal of the American Medical Association*) *Internal Medicine* (posted online April 15, 2013), investigators determined the frequency and category of dietary supplements recalled from January 1, 2004 through December 19, 2012. Within that period, 237 such supplements were recalled citing a "reasonable probability that the use of or exposure to the product will cause serious adverse health consequences or death". Of the 237 products recalled, sixty-four (27 percent) were found to be in the weight loss category. It should be noted that while no adverse events associated with these products were reported, it was concern about the *probability* of such an event that prompted the FDA to act. If it is primarily concerns about death that stirs the FDA into action, the mere fact that a product does not perform as advertised will probably leave them sitting on their hands.

On the subject of consequences, I assume I am not putting myself in legal jeopardy by calling attention to these fraudulent practices. If the grocery store tabloids can take a scorched earth approach to their reporting on public figures, surely I can cast a critical eye in the direction of the weight loss industry. For the industry and their defenders, ours is a capitalistic society that many argue operates best in the absence of unnecessary governmental intervention. The marketplace will see to itself, so they might say, by having the ultimate need to respond to the wants of the consumer.

It is plain to see the weight loss industry is in fact listening to the public. They have heard the call for products that would bring to an end the suffering of the overweight. In response to that call, vast arrays of slickly marketed products are available for purchase both online and through brick and mortar stores. However, as has been discussed, the products fall short in delivering on their promise. Therefore, while it may be fair to say that the industry is *listening*, it is no less fair to say that the products they're producing to address the demands are in the main ineffective. If the marketplace were truly effective at policing itself, the majority of these products would no longer be available. As it relates to the weight loss industry, the rules of supply and demand do not seem to apply, for their supply surely fails to address the demand.

It appears that the industry has learned where diet supplements are concerned the key is not to build a better mousetrap; it is simply to build one. For that matter, the particular trap need not even be of their own creation. As have many in the past, one can simply remove it from someone else's shelf, dust it off, put on a pretty label (perhaps featuring an impossibly thin model), make a few outlandish claims regarding its potential, and it will live anew.

Chapter 7

On Raising Weight
Appropriate Children

As an introduction to this chapter, I will admit that I am not a father; I have no children of my own. I cannot pretend to understand the difficulty being a parent poses or know the joy it brings. You who are parents will question my authority to make recommendations on any subject connected to rearing children. However, as it relates to managing the weight of children, I believe parenthood is not a necessary prerequisite. Still, I encourage you in this instance, as in all matters, to maintain a healthy sense of skepticism, without it, one cannot hope to reach accurate conclusions. If at any point during this chapter you find the need to say, "That's easy for you to say; you're not a father", then have at it.

The first and perhaps most salient point is that children, particularly infants, are not merely smaller versions of ourselves. Children are unique unto themselves with distinct anatomy, physiology, and personal care requirements, which we must take into account when providing for their needs. One of their anatomical distinctions is that they are skeletally immature. From an orthopedic perspective, this makes them vulnerable to a list of injuries common to those in their stage of life. Beyond orthopedics, there are differences in airway size that put children at increased risk for choking. Their greater skin to body size ratio, referred to as body surface area (BSA), leaves them more susceptible to heat illness and to injury through the absorption of toxins. Owing to their decreased muscle tone and the increased elasticity of their rib cage, the organs within their chest and abdomen are less protected against blunt force trauma and are, therefore, more vulnerable to injury associated with such trauma.

This is by no means an exhaustive list of the anatomic differences that exist between them and us. It is instead a small sampling through which I have attempted to illustrate the fact that while children are a product of us, they are not us, at least as it pertains to these measures. A similarly lengthy list of physiologic differences could be offered, but for the purposes of this book I hope it is adequate to say that they exist. It is truly outside the scope of this book (and for that matter its author), to delve into these weighty scholarly issues. The one distinction I will discuss relates to differences in the size and number of fat cells present in the adult and the child and what becomes of those fat cells when weight is lost or gained. Because this topic is so central to the conversation on weight management, it may in fact be ground zero in the fight against obesity and overweightness for people of all ages.

Let us first dispense with the notion that fat serves no useful purpose in the human body; that it is nothing more than a means of storing excess energy. While it is that, it is also an important player in a number of chemical processes. Its role in releasing selected hormones into the bloodstream has only recently been discovered. Among other things, these hormones affect appetite, insulin sensitivity, immune response, as well as reproductive function. With these various functions, fat participates in the processes that serve to maintain a stable internal environment, a condition referred to in high school science as homeostasis. When operating in the presence of such an environment, the human body performs like a well-oiled machine. However, when that environment is stressed or disturbed, which can occur in the case of supernormal fat stores, the body may become desensitized to the hormones and fail to respond to the messages they send. Some researchers have linked those disturbances tied to increased fat stores with heart disease, high blood pressure, diabetes, osteoarthritis, cancer, and other chronic diseases.

Knowing that fat cells are active participants in the chemical dance we call life, may serve to lessen concern when you learn that at birth we each have some five- to ten billion fat cells on board. The exact number appears to have no connection to an established family history of obesity. Put another way, children of obese parents have not been found to have significantly more fat cells at birth than do the children of average-weighted parents. So I have to ask, is obesity a product of nurture or nature? In all probability, it is some combination of the two; however, what is certain is that obese children are far more likely to grow into obese adults than are children of healthy weight. Also certain is that childhood obesity has become a leading health concern having tripled from 5 percent in the 1970s to 15 percent in the first decade of this millennium. The message here is both clear and chilling; either we assert control over what is being referred to as an emerging pandemic, or face a healthcare crisis the likes of which we have not seen.

To understand the physiology of obesity, let's go back to the fat cell. As mentioned in the previous paragraph, we begin life with a number said to hover around ten billion. Recent research suggests that that number can be added to during the years leading up to early adulthood. At that age and beyond, the number of fat cells appears to remain constant. Therefore, when adults gain weight, we are simply adding to the volume of an existing cell whereas children are actually increasing the number of those cells. These increases can find upward of thirty billion fat cells in a healthy adult, seventy-five billion amassed in an overweight individual, and two hundred billion or more among the severely obese; all other things being equal, the greater the number of fat cells the greater the potential to store and carry fat. If it is within our ability to do so, should we not endeavor to control the number of fat cells we lay down? If I may answer my own question, definitively yes!

As to the role genetics may play in the development of obesity, I think even in the absence of strong corroboration it is reasonable to conclude there is a linkage. As in most questions related to the human body, I would, however, hedge my bets. Our owner's manual is far from complete. What we know of this machine remains a moving target. That about which we were convinced yesterday we could refute tomorrow. Whatever role genetics may play, I would not want it to become a rationalization for quitting, for throwing your hands up, and saying that the die has been cast. Tell me if you've heard this before - nothing about weight loss will be easy!

Accepting that weight loss is a challenge, if through our efforts we can help our children to avoid this fate, surely they will be far better off for it. Part of that process requires that we ourselves pattern healthy behaviors. Much discussed in recent years is the question of whether athletes act, wittingly or otherwise, as role models in the lives of children, and if so, to what extent. Whichever side of the debate you happen to take, that which is undeniably true is the preeminent role that parents play in shaping the attitudes, beliefs, and behaviors of their children. Recognizing the sway parents wield in the lives of their children should serve as motivation to those who want to create lasting positive associations with food and exercise. With that as our goal, we cannot make poor food choices and expect our children won't do likewise. We cannot demonstrate disordered eating habits and think our children won't behave similarly. We cannot refrain from exercise if we expect our children to embrace it.

On the latter point, I believe it is a child's natural inclination to play. They are young colts (or fillies as the case may be) running from the moment it is possible to do so. It is only when we impose our needs that their interest seems to wane. We judge, evaluate, critique, and score. We set guidelines, establish rules, create boundaries, and implement performance standards. In short, we do everything to nullify the joy and steal away the spontaneity that is at the heart of childhood movement. Instead of asking children to participate in the games and activities we choose, we should encourage them to do those things that bring them happiness. Let them experience success as they define it. In the interest of helping our children stay on the path leading to good health, we should make it our mission to nurture in them a positive relationship with physical activity. Having fostered such a relationship, you can trust your children will find their way to organized sports if and when they are ready to do so. Until such time, allow them to do what children do.

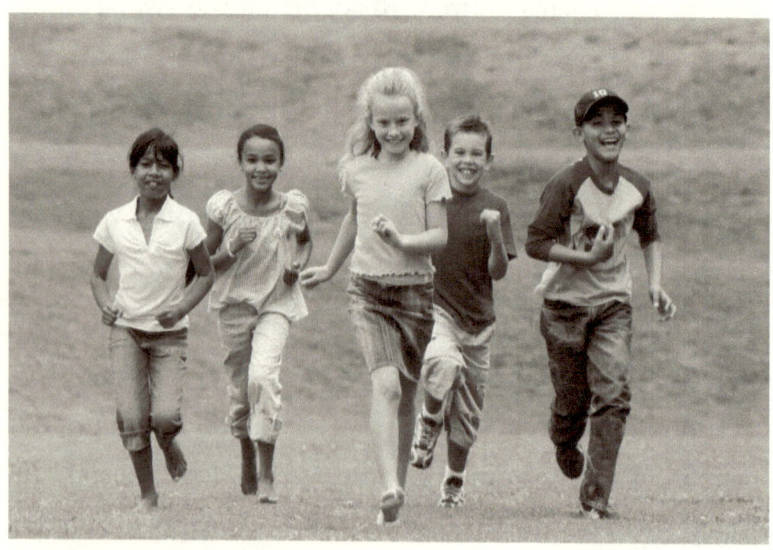

Video games and social media have the potential to steal time away from meaningful physical activity. To the extent necessary, encourage children to get outdoors and play.

What children also do is eat fast food. According to one study (Effects of fast-food consumption on energy intake and diet quality among children in a national household survey, Bowman SA, Gortmaker SL, et al, *Pediatrics* 2004 Jan; 113 [1 Pt 1], 112-8.), everyday nearly one third of American children aged four to nineteen eat fast food, a fivefold increase since 1970. Without getting into the whys and wherefores, this is simply not sustainable. With this comment, I hear a chorus of "That's easy for you to say," but the parents among you must act to limit the role that the fast-food industry plays in the feeding of your children.

I understand what motivates the choice - it is cheap, it is convenient, and it is often the path of least resistance. After having battled through your own workday, you return home to contemplate dinner. You could poll the family to determine what they would like to eat, which would likely yield multiple disparate options. Alternatively, you could prepare a meal without consulting the family, which would surely leave some dissatisfied, or you could pile everyone in the car and drive to the fast-food chain of choice, which in itself might create some controversy. Once you've committed to a restaurant (here I use the term advisedly), all is right with the world. You might even use it as leverage for the kids to do their homework, or take a bath, or write that overdue thank you note. Whatever the case, you are instantly in their good graces because your children don't care about what is good for them; they only care about what is good.

Unfortunately the fast-food industry has invested countless dollars in an effort to understand children's culinary proclivities, if I can use such an expression when discussing fast-food, and more importantly, how best to market to them. Make no mistake, it is to them that the industry markets. While some municipalities have attempted to put an end to toy giveaways as part of meals targeted to children, the practice is still widespread throughout the country. Truth be told, even if the practice were to end today, I believe that the industry has carved such a deep and abiding niche in the American culture it would have little effect on their bottom line.

Fast-food is here to stay. As evidence of their strength, revenues have grown from six billion dollars in 1970 to one hundred sixty billion dollars in 2012. According to Eric Schlosser (*Fast-Food Nation*) "Americans now spend more money on fast food than on higher education, personal computers, computer software, or new cars. They spend more on fast-food than on movies, books, magazines, newspapers, videos, and recorded music – combined."

Against that backdrop, parents must wage their own wars to win back control of their children's food choices. With that as their aim, those parents must work to eliminate fast-food from their own diet. For some, that will not be an easy assignment. Many are already well ensconced in the fast-food lifestyle that prizes foods, spanning the range from sweet to savory with little room for, or regard to, healthy offerings. If not for themselves but for their children, parents must resolve to end their relationship with fast-food.

At this point, you must be asking yourself, surely, he does not mean to eliminate fast-food? While I did previously mention moderation, and generally accept it as a principle guiding our eating habits, I believe where children are concerned, it becomes an especially slippery slope. In a study conducted at the National Taiwan University (Childhood obesity and unhappiness: the influence of soft drink and fast-food consumption, Hung-Hao Chang, Rodolfo M Nayga. *Journal of Happiness Studies*, 2009), researchers found that not only are moms who turn to fast-food more likely to have children who do, but that those children who regularly consume fast-food, while more likely to be overweight, are also less likely to be unhappy. Extrapolating that same data to our children would have to give one concern over the power that fast-food may hold in their lives. If children equate fast food with happiness, separating them from it may lead to tension at home.

Do you then make a conscious effort to keep children away from these establishments knowing that at some point they will celebrate a birthday party or other occasion there? I would say it is a virtual impossibility to insulate them from fast-food. Since we cannot and probably should not do that, we must explain to them that it is appropriate only on the rare occasion. We must work to make them understand the important role that food plays in providing us with the nutrients necessary to function at our best. I have no doubt that it would be a difficult sell, and again, as one who has no children, I could not begin to tell you how that conversation should sound, but I suspect it would have to be repeated on many occasions before it takes root.

I was raised in a different America, not better or worse, simply different. During my youth, my father worked and my mother stayed at home and attended to my siblings and myself. In our household, breakfast was provided, lunch was prepared and sent with us to school, and dinner was eaten at the table. We rarely deviated from this pattern. Fast-food restaurants existed, but were far less ubiquitous. My memory is of meals prepared with balance, most including vegetables that my sister would push around her plate until she was finally excused from the table.

Times have certainly changed. Today, households in which both parents work have surpassed those that predominated when I was a child. In a 2000 Census Bureau report, 51 percent of married couples with children both worked. With both parents working to support the family, fewer than 40 percent with children under eighteen had dinner together seven nights a week. Within this brave New World, fast food has become an option far too often exercised and we feel the affect. It is no accident that our obesity rates rose in lockstep with the revenues of the fast-food industry. The industry has gotten fat, in a financial sense, at our expense while we have merely gotten progressively fatter in the literal sense.

In an attempt to illustrate the adverse health effects of the fast-food diet, independent filmmaker Morgan Spurlock subjected himself to a thirty-day period of all fast-food fare. Chronicled in the 2004 documentary, *Super Size Me*, Spurlock's self-imposed conditions required that he eat each of his three meals at a McDonald's restaurant and that he do so in an uninterrupted fashion for 30 consecutive days. Although he could not specifically request it, on those occasions when he was asked if he wanted to supersize (increasing the portion size of each item selected) the meal, he did so as another stipulation of the examination.

At the conclusion of his thirty-day trial, Spurlock noted changes in his blood chemistry, mood, and sexual function, but most germane to this book was his twenty-four-and-a-half pound weight gain brought on by his average daily consumption of five thousand calories. The diet he put himself through would not be typical for even the most ardent fast-food aficionado, but the after-effects do point to an urgent need to address our fast-food obsession. It is a trend we must reverse, so why not let it be at the expense of the fast-food industry that has for too long profited at our expense? For your benefit and that of your children I encourage you to dial back your support.

Chapter 8

Back to You

In the preceding few chapters, we veered off course slightly by glancing at some issues that may not be directly related to your situation. Unless you're a retired athlete, one about to retire, or the parent of a child dealing with its own troubles related to weight, you may have found little value in the information presented. However, behind the specific populations discussed is the underlying theme of energy balance.

Remembering that I am but one of thousands who have written on the subject, how does my position square with those expressed by others? I hope it will not surprise you to learn there is no unanimity of opinion. In fact, with respect to calorie restriction, some argue loudly against it as a weight loss strategy. Those who do, claim it has a poor track record where sustained weight loss is concerned. They contend that starving yourself during one meal may cause you to overcompensate at the next. If true, I would suggest what they describe is not an example of calorie restriction at all. Starving and binging are merely other forms of disordered eating. What I have advocated and continue to advocate for is a moderate but consistent decrease in the amount of food we consume throughout the course of the day. What I have suggested could not reasonably be thought of as starvation. One of my stated goals is to assist you in establishing, or reestablishing, a healthy and sustainable relationship with the food you eat. Starving and binging is neither healthy, nor is it sustainable in the long-term.

The less obtrusive a change is made to be, the easier it is to internalize, to sustain. This is particularly true when taking on a challenge the likes of weight loss. Statistics would have you believe that in this task you are up against it. When compared with those who have fallen short of their goals, we could count on one hand those who have succeeded. Accepting this assertion as true, at least in relative terms, the next question becomes, what will you do to set yourself apart, to succeed where others have failed, and where perhaps you yourself have failed in the past? It starts by believing that you are bigger than the test before you, that regardless the number who have fallen, you will prevail. Yes, weight loss requires that your energy intake be exceeded by your energy expenditures, but this knowledge will only take you so far.

Willpower is the capacity of a person to pick a course and stick to it by exercising control over those impulses that might otherwise lead you astray. In the matter of weight loss, willpower reigns supreme. Doubters might say that if you had willpower, you wouldn't find yourself in your present predicament. This is often said in an accusatory fashion as in, "She will never lose weight; she has no willpower".

For some among you that may be true. I don't mean to suggest that it is a strength of character issue but rather one of impulse control. Increasingly, those who have great difficulty restraining their feeding behaviors are finding help, not through nutritional counseling, but through mental health counseling. Challenging prevailing public thought that obesity and overweight are conditions of sloth; mental health professionals are tackling it as an "impulse control disorder". For what percentage of the more than two hundred million overweight or obese Americans would such treatment be in order? The question is impossible to answer with certainty, but regardless the number, I believe a great many of this country's overweight are capable of walking back, both literally and figuratively, their weight, and their BMI's. Are you such a person, someone who has fond, albeit distant memories of being at a weight appropriate for your frame? Have you simply strayed too far from the path you once walked and need help to find your way back? If this describes your situation, I urge you to stay on this journey. Your problems are not insurmountable. You can overcome your obstacles and reach your aims. The information presented thus far, and that which follows, I offer up with your aims in mind. It is my intention to clear the brush that has obscured the path leading you to, or back to, a healthier way of living.

Every day we are asked to make choices, to decide issues both large and small. Our choices can determine what we do today or how we spend the rest of our lives. Even seemingly insignificant choices can yield decisions that have far-reaching consequences. Your choices related to diet and exercise serve as excellent illustrations of the point. Whether you're planning for your own meals or those of your family, each day you're made to decide, what will today's meals consist of? Taken separately, you'd have a difficult time convincing anyone that such a decision is life altering. A single meal, regardless its composition, does not provide much insight into your nutrition habits. However, to the extent that any one meal is an accurate reflection of your preferred food choices, the content of that meal becomes more meaningful and the decision to choose it more significant.

While I do not necessarily subscribe to the notion that you are what you eat, I do believe that what you eat provides evidence of your tastes and in some cases, your nutritional weaknesses. To better understand the pattern of your eating habits, I typically recommend that you chart your food and drink consumption for one to two months. When doing so, you must be completely truthful in your reporting of the description, quantity, and timing of each item eaten or imbibed. Because you will be using this information for your own purposes, you should not withhold items for fear of being judged. In the case of this reporting, accuracy is the watchword.

Living Life Lean Daily Food Log

Date	Time	Food Item	Approximate Calorie Count	Reflection (Before, During, After)

Keeping in mind that no single aberrant meal is by itself destructive, the purpose of this exercise is not to call attention to the odd transgression. It is rather the purpose to look at what is typical or normal for you in an effort to establish your common fare. Since mood, attitude, or circumstance often intervenes in our choices, particularly as they relate to food, I also suggest that some reference to it be included in your recording of any item eaten (reflection). For instance, if you were to indicate that in association with consuming a quart of ice cream you were angry secondary to a conflict on the job, it would suggest that at least in this instance, you used food in a maladaptive way as a coping device.

When in possession of this information, you can better determine the breadth of your difficulties tied to nutrition. Laid out in black and white it is not possible to escape what are likely to be some surprising but obvious conclusions. Frequently reported by those who have charted their eating habits is dismay about the discovery that fruits and vegetables were so underrepresented, or that fast-food made up a larger percentage of meals taken, or how often junk foods had found their way into the diet.

To refer to any of these realizations as discoveries might seem like an example of poor word choice; after all you consciously selected each food you ate. Still how many of us remember what we had for dinner last night, let alone a week or two in the past? Our memory regarding diet quickly becomes fogged by time. We can't hope to correct that which we don't recall. Through this charting we're able to summon forth all of our gastronomic activity for evaluation. What we are attempting to do is establish a pattern of eating. Within that pattern we would hope to learn what reasonable adjustments we could make to reduce calorie intake in order to better position ourselves to lose weight.

When reliably completed, the chart also provides other useful information. From it, we can discern the distribution of calories consumed throughout the course of the day, and the relative macronutrient composition of those calories. Stated more plainly, what percentage of your calories come from carbohydrates, proteins and fats, and if that composition is appropriate to your needs. Where fats are concerned, are they largely saturated or the lesser objectionable polyunsaturated or monounsaturated fats? Indeed the latter two are not only less objectionable, they are also thought to reduce the risk of heart disease and type 2 diabetes and are therefore potentially helpful fats.

Regarding your carbohydrate intake, does your record indicate it is principally in the form of the simple, or are the more advantageous complex better represented? On this matter, confusion abounds. Many of today's more commercially popular diet plans condemn carbohydrates as a blight on the American diet. Just as we cannot lump all fats into one category, neither can we do so with carbohydrates.

Sure, simple carbohydrates such as table sugar, soft drinks, cookies, candy, syrups and the like are primary evildoers in diet related health issues, but to label all carbohydrates as villains is not just inaccurate, it's patently false.

As the brain and body's preferred energy source, carbohydrates are meant to constitute a majority of your daily calorie intake. Falling somewhere in the range of 45-65 percent of your total calories, carbohydrates play critical roles in a multitude of physiologic functions and as a result, you should make no attempt to limit their intake. I make this comment with regard to complex carbohydrates specifically because it is a fair point that we Americans consume far too many simple carbohydrates and for reasons other than simply weight, we should endeavor to purge them, at least the worst offenders, from our diet.

Recalling our earlier discussion of nutrient density, it is important, particularly when dieting, that we extract the maximum nutrient value from the calories we consume. We have precious little room for foods that return nothing on the investment. In this case, the investment I reference is the one you make in your good health. The investment you've made, or are making, is less a monetary one than it is one of effort and energy. The return you seek is in the form of decreased weight and increased general health. Ramping up your consumption of fruits and vegetables is one sure way to earn this end. Note the use of the word *earn* in the previous sentence. I've always thought it was an easy matter for those of us who enjoy fruits and vegetables to recommend them to those who don't. Pound for pound, they deliver a big nutrient punch carrying large concentrations of vitamins, minerals and the too often underappreciated fiber, all at an enticingly low calorie cost. Still, if you can't bring yourself to put them on your plate, let alone in your mouth their nutrient value is effectively zero.

If you share former President George H. W. Bush's revulsion of broccoli, if you are like the *Seinfeld* character Newman, find it to be a vile weed then the knowledge that it contains healthy concentrations of vitamins A, B complex, C, E and K means nothing to you. The fact this vegetable is rich in several vital minerals, likewise, does little to persuade you. If your solution to the problem is to ladle on massive quantities of melted cheese, whatever you've gained by eating the broccoli is more than offset by the equally massive increase in calories coming primarily in the form of saturated fat.

The good news amid the bad is that broccoli is not your only option. The produce section of your neighborhood grocery store is chock-full of alternatives that rise up out of the earth to meet your nutrient needs. I will stipulate that some of you would rather eat the dirt out of which they rise than some of the vegetables themselves, but I am confident that even the most over particular among you will find options that suit your tastes.

An excellent, albeit for some unpalatable, alternative is the salad. Unpalatable, I suspect because for many it amounts to a radical departure from your normal eating pattern. If this forms the basis for your opposition, I understand. I have attempted to nudge you in the direction of healthier choices; the salad may amount to more of a full-body check. But if you'll allow room for it, the salad can become a way station on the road between where you are in terms of your eating habits and where we ultimately hope you'll be.

Consider this, today's salad, for better or worse, is not your mother's salad. While it may continue to include some leafy vegetables, its list of other ingredients has been broadly expanded. For those who have difficulty warming up to the notion of eating a salad made exclusively from vegetables then perhaps the addition of some other ingredients will work to tamp down your aversion. As a rule, I discourage the practice of adding fatty meats and cheeses to a salad, but in the interest of transitioning you to a place where it is possible to support the inclusion of salad as a meal choice then go ahead sprinkle a little cheese or crumble on a piece of bacon. If this small concession is what it takes to bring vegetables into your life in a more significant way, do it. I'm betting that over time you will grow to enjoy the other components of your salad sufficiently so as to allow for the eventual elimination of the more artery-challenging elements.

Constructing Your Salad

In one form or another, most every country and culture has an equivalent to what we generically refer to as salad. Prepared using ingredients endemic to the particular corner of the globe from which they originate, salads come in a nearly infinite variety. I suspect those Americans who tend to view salads in a negative light have not exposed themselves to the offerings of other cultures or even to the full array of options available to them here.

A side salad served at a local restaurant is frequently little more than a few assorted lettuce leaves, but it is such a mix that many folks conjure up when they give thought to the odious salad. I believe salads need not be odious at all. In fact, if you seek variety in your food choices there may be no better option than salad. The salad you create is limited only by the extent of your imagination. Fruits and vegetables, nuts and seeds, herbs and spices, meat, fish, poultry, rice, pasta, beans, sprouts, mushrooms and more. Chopped, wedged, shredded, diced, minced, julienned, pickled, some ingredients cooked, and others served raw; the rule regarding salad construction is that there is no rule at all. Experiment to your heart's delight, find that combination or those combinations that appeal best to you and write your own definition of the term salad.

Controversial as it will always be, the United States Department of Agriculture's (USDA) Food Guide Pyramid presently recommends that adults consume two to four servings of fruit and three to five servings of vegetables daily. Unfortunately, many of us fall woefully short of these numbers. The inclusion of salad into your diet can quickly fill the void where those recommendations are concerned. Although this is not principally a book on the science of nutrition, it would be wrong to ignore what science tells us about the known health benefits of a diet rich in fruits and vegetables.

Undisputed is their role in bringing much-needed fiber to our diets. Not to be too indelicate here, but fiber increases the motility or movement of our waste through the colon that works to prevent constipation that is a common consequence of a diet high in fat. Additionally, and of great importance to the calorie conscious, is the fact that their generally low calorie cost allows us to eat a larger volume and therefore come to a feeling of fullness at a point much earlier than we might if we were to eat a more calorie-dense alternative. It is a pet supposition of mine that it is not only the volume of these foods, but the time and energy needed to consume them, which contributes to the sense of satiety. Referring particularly to the raw vegetables commonly found in salads, there is a significant investment in time required to grind them up to a size and consistency suitable for swallowing. The time spent bringing these foods to that state allow us the opportunity to become aware of our progress toward fullness rather than to be struck by it at the conclusion of the meal (see Thanksgiving dinner).

My suppositions aside, researchers in the field of nutrition continue to investigate the part that plant foods play in health and disease. Although conclusive statements are yet to be made available, research increasingly supports a linkage between the regular consumption of fruits and vegetables and the decreased risk of a variety of diseases up to and including cancer. When confronted with all of this information, if you remain on the fence where fruits and vegetables are concerned then think about this, beneficial as this category of foods is, we have much more to learn. Of particular interest is the role of phytonutrients or phytochemicals that are found in great abundance in plant foods. It is reasonable to presume that these foods may be more advantageous than we currently know. The long and short of it is that whatever you hope to accomplish through weight loss, you have no better partner than fruits and vegetables.

If you understand and appreciate this information, but still can't bring yourself to eat vegetables, I will make one last plea in support of salad. By bringing the variety of tastes and textures together on a single plate you create a delightful interplay that has a tendency to overpower any elements that singly you might find noxious. Even the vile weed broccoli can find a place in your diet when balanced against the spiciness of a radish, or the sweetness of a red pepper, or the nutty flavor of an avocado (okay, not a vegetable but you get the idea). Regardless how strongly I implore, some of you will never find your way to the consistent inclusion of salads. However, I am certain of one thing, for those who do, salad will become a weight loss game changer in your effort to shed pounds.

Salad Dressing

You can't discuss salad without including some reference to salad dressing. For some people, a salad is not complete until they have ladled an amount of dressing on top. I've used the term *ladled* here intentionally to describe the manner in which the dressing is applied to the salad. Whatever the volume of dressing the ladle carries know it is typically well beyond the recommended two tablespoon serving size. Even if no more than two tablespoons were added the affect would be to bring an additional 100-200 calories (the majority of which comes in the form of fat) to the salad individually and the meal collectively. More likely, the dressing added exceeds two tablespoons by a sizeable margin and the calories ingested increase accordingly. To avoid those otherwise empty calories, I would encourage you to consider eating your salad sans dressing. For those nauseated by the notion of a "dressingless" salad, a slightly less objectionable recommendation would be to put your dressing in a small cup or bowl and place it alongside your salad. By doing so, you could then insert the tines of your fork into the dressing ahead of spearing some item or items from the salad. In this way, with each bite, you can appreciate some of the dressing's flavor without taking on a significant calorie hit.

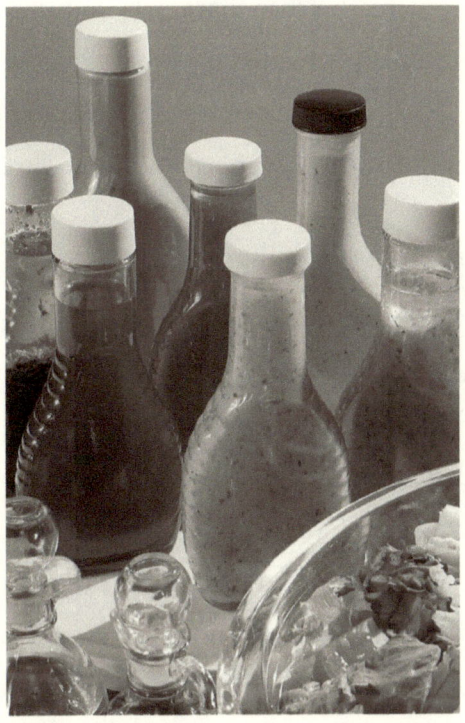

If you were to do nothing more than feature salads in your diet, change will come. If you simultaneously step up your personal exercise load, you're on your way. To monitor your exercise activity, I would ask that you log those activities in the same way I advised regarding your diet. Alternatively, there are numerous devices available for purchase that accomplish this same purpose without requiring you to put pencil to paper or fingers to a keyboard. Regardless the vehicle, the objective is to see increases, documented changes in the energy expended during the course of your day. In contrast to the diet diary, whose purpose you will recall is to establish your dietary preferences and patterns, the exercise log is meant as a written reminder of what you have done and a source of motivation encouraging you to do more.

Yes, it is true, you don't have to be an athlete or even athletic to ask more of yourself physically. It's not about slam dunks or homeruns. It's about movement. Dropping weight is predicated upon it; it and, of course, the much discussed decreased consumption. In a world increasingly devoid of logic, nothing could be more logical. Yet we continue to turn to pills, supplements, and shakes hoping against hope that in them we will find a simple path to slimming, one that does not inconvenience us in any way since that appears to be our primary objective - to lose weight while we continue to do what we've done all along.

Living Life Lean Weekly Activity Log

Date	Activity	Duration (Time)	Intensity (Easy, Medium, Hard)	Reflection (Before, During, After)

I cannot confidently argue that no one has ever known success from the use of these products. My considered opinion is, those who have achieved some measure of success have done so principally through the concepts thus far outlined. If you've employed some of these strategies in concert with a supplement, that supplement will frequently be credited with any success achieved. This is especially true when a celebrity endorser or TV doctor touts the product. Our vulnerability to people we perceive as knowledgeable or influential is well preyed upon by all manner of industry, not the least of which is the weight loss industry.

For those who sell their influence, their celebrity for personal gain without thought to how their actions may harm others, to them I say go in shame. However, I will reserve my most stern rebuke for the doctors turned TV personalities who, for the sake of audience share, promote products and practices that have no basis in science. To those men and women who swore an oath to "do no harm," I am especially critical. As part of that same oath, doctors swear that into each house they enter, they go expressly for the benefit of the patient. Today, a small number of those oath takers enter our homes via our TV screens, but unlike the physicians of yore, their purpose appears more in line with entertainment than edification, more about sensationalism than good sense.

Fame is a powerful drug. In pursuit of it, many have abandoned their own ideals and those of their profession without the slightest evidence of compunction. If you are among the people who take your lead from those in the media, I urge you to exercise extreme caution and do as my father always suggested, "consider the source". Of course, you might think that doctors would be reliable sources for information on health and wellness, but as I have attempted to illustrate, even they can become corrupted by their baser instincts. Regardless your interests, when exploring any subject, choose your sources wisely.

In my case, I typically turn to those who have significant experience working in the area about which I have questions. This is not to say I don't value education because I certainly do. However, in my experience, education merely qualifies one to perform a particular occupation. It is in so performing that the real learning occurs.

Take for instance Dr. Fred Goldman. At one hundred and one years old, Dr. Goldman has been practicing medicine for seventy-seven years. During the span of his practice, you would have to imagine Dr. Goldman has learned a thing or two about the human body in general and his in particular. When asked about his secrets to a long life, the doctor claims he has none. He hasn't a clue why he has lived as long as he has. In answer to a specific question regarding exercise Dr. Goldman indicated that in his mind "it is overrated". He does not and has not exercised in the traditional sense but he does keep moving which, he says, is his workout.

Dr. Goldman's comments point to the importance of lifestyle. To the extent that he has an explanation for the length of his life, he credits movement. He has made movement, either consciously or unconsciously, a central tenet of his life. If there is a single take away from the life he has led, it is that movement (at least as he defines it) may be enough. However, that movement must find its way into our lives every day, not as a means of offsetting a dietary transgression – I ate that, therefore I must do this – instead it must become part and parcel of who we are. I don't know how else to say it; we cannot choose to be inactive and expect to be trim, the terms sedentary and fit are mutually exclusive.

Although I know any diet plan or program can trot out, or failing that, conjure up their respective successes as models of what can be achieved, I would like to offer concrete examples of what two men did achieve by recommitting themselves to movement and exercise.

A Career Change Begets A Life Change

At forty-five Stan stood five feet seven and weighed a robust two hundred twelve pounds. Like many men Stan's age, his weight had accrued during the nearly thirty years since he graduated high school, a slim and svelte eighteen-year-old. No longer the lithe-bodied athlete he had once been, he had succumbed to the demands that the life of a married father of two requires.

Having spent a good number of those thirty years as a trader on the Pacific Stock Exchange, Stan freely selected from the calorie laden fast-foods that were as much a part of the traders' day as were stock quotes themselves. Conscious of his weight change, Stan did little to resist the inexorable slide into what he felt was on some level his destiny. Mind you, he did not bear this destiny alone. Surrounded by men of similar heft, Stan imagined most men his age either wrestled with their weight or accepted its increases as a consequence of the aging process. Content to carry on with the life he was leading, Stan had no grand designs to alter his current course; as often happens, the coming change of course would be dictated by events outside his control.

The layoff came first. Precipitated by technological changes that made his job obsolete, the layoff left Stan unemployed for the first time in his adult life. Although his wife worked, the family had grown accustomed to the lifestyle that two incomes provided. Seeking to maintain that lifestyle Stan quickly set out in pursuit of other opportunities. Regrettably, after months of sustained effort, he continued to be among the unemployed.

Frustrated by his inability to find a new situation, Stan enrolled in classes at a nearby university. Upon completion the particular course of study on which he had embarked would qualify Stan to work with athletes as a healthcare provider. During the course of that accreditation, the other shoe dropped.

It was early spring, a time for renewal and rebirth, and Stan a long time soccer fan was participating in an adult league match. During the second half of the match, an opponent elbowed Stan in the ribs. Though undeniably sore, he gave it little thought believing it would pass in a day or two. A week later, not only had the soreness not passed, it had intensified. Urged by his wife, Stan sought the counsel of a physician. Although the physician's diagnosis was benign enough, he took the extra step and ordered a scan to rule out other possibilities. The scan detected an unrelated cancerous growth.

A spiritual man, Stan took this startling news in stride. He reasoned that were it not for the layoff and the unsuccessful job search that followed, he might not have come to a place where the cancer would have been discovered in a timely fashion. As it was, doctors removed the growth, Stan completed his studies, and soon thereafter found gainful employment.

Now employed in his new field, Stan concluded that for personal and professional reasons, he needed to lose weight.

While working at the Pacific Stock Exchange he would have given little thought to his weight; however, as one responsible for the care and counsel of athletes, it was no longer tenable. He felt that he could not encourage athletes to eat properly if he did not set a positive example. Stan rightly concluded that where athletes were concerned, the hypocrisy inherent in the "Do as I say not as I do" attitude would not fly.

Supremely motivated, Stan met this challenge head-on. With adjustments to his diet and exercise alone, in three months' time he had shed twenty pounds, and eight months later twenty more. More significant still, is the fact that two years after having embarked on this journey, not a single pound of that lost weight has returned.

Without pharmaceutical assistance, without crash dieting, without hours spent at the gym, Stan achieved his weight loss goals. In order to do so, he scaled back his eating and increased his activity. Specifically, he purchased a treadmill and used in with great consistency. He chose running as the catalyst for his weight reduction. Although he would not describe his pace as blistering, he was unshakable in his commitment to running.

Be committed to whatever form or forms of activity you choose to engage in. Finding time for activity on a consistent basis is a necessary precondition to losing weight and preventing its return.

From Beer to Activity

Jorge came to the United States by way of Mexico at the not-so-tender age of thirty-nine. Like those I referenced in chapter 1, Jorge came to this country in hopes of improving his lot and his luck, of increasing his opportunities to achieve success in the way that he defined it.

When Jorge arrived, he was not a lean man. Neither, I should say, was he grossly overweight. Like many on either side of the border (Mexico has recently surpassed the United States as the most obese country), Jorge knew that he could stand to lose some weight. Unfortunately, during his first few years in America, he only added to his girth.

According to Jorge, it wasn't the variety of food he ate that found him in such a state - he continued to eat the foods most familiar to him. It was instead the volume of food that was behind Jorge's weight gain - that and a fondness for alcohol, beer in particular. As an answer to his own dilemma, Jorge made what for him was the difficult decision to cut out the beer. He further resolved to be mindful of the quantity of food he was consuming and to find some room in his life for activity. As it pertains to this latter consideration, Jorge exerted himself during his workday, leaving him well spent by the time his day was done. However, like every other successful dieter, Jorge believed he couldn't achieve his goal of losing weight unless he was to make a conscious effort to do more.

Never having read anything on the subject of dieting, he instinctively knew that exercise would help him with his mission. Not a runner like Stan, Jorge chose to walk. And walk he did. Within two months, Jorge was walking an hour per day, five days per week. At five months into the process, Jorge had lost twenty pounds. On the one-year anniversary of the start of his quest, he had lost a total of thirty pounds.

When speaking to Jorge about his success, he confided that cutting the beer out of his diet played the largest role. I, on the other hand, believe his commitment to consistent exercise was no less important. I say that not knowing how much beer Jorge had been drinking. On that subject he shared no details, but the empty calories consumed in the form of alcohol could easily account for the added weight. If one were otherwise in calorie balance, then dropping alcohol, whatever the form, would at least cease any further weight gain. The weight loss in this scenario would only occur through changes in diet and exercise. For Jorge, and I suspect for most, how the weight comes off is less important than whether it comes off.

Losing weight requires the steely-eyed determination that both Stan and Jorge possessed during the course of their respective journeys. Minus an unwavering sense of self-confidence, a belief in your ability to achieve the desired end, your best intentions will be for naught. I am not one who believes that we are each capable of accomplishing anything that we want in life. The evidence against it is strong. However, I do believe those who want to can lose weight. Though Stan and Jorge may be shining examples of that, they are by no means alone. Others have known the sense of accomplishment that comes from achieving this goal. For most, it comes about in a similar way – a defining moment, an event that crystallizes the need to act and the actions themselves. Specifically, correcting disordered eating habits and making room for movement in one's life. Do this for yourself. Start now.

Chapter 9

~

Optimal Health Encapsulated

I must say the idea of sheathing our every need in a pill fits perfectly into the modern American lifestyle. For the benefit of our convenience we have pills for nearly every occasion. If its sleep you need, there is a pill. If that pill leaves you groggy, we have pills to clear the fog. If your life finds you anxious, there is a pill to calm you down, or if depressed, pills to lift you up. If hair loss is your problem, don't fret, there is a pill. Is pain your issue? For that, there are many pills. Oh, and should those pain pills leave you constipated, yes, there are pills for that as well.

We are a nation of pill takers, an appetite developed during our infancy. Every illness or distress we suffer as children is in some way countered by a pill; often given with a mother's love expressed in warm and tender tones. There can be no surer path to dependency.

In a country that so openly embraces pills as the answer to a great many of its ills, can we be surprised when pills are promoted as the answer to our nutritional deficiencies? Should your diet fail to provide you with the nutrients you require, don't bother adjusting your diet because those nutrients are available in the form of a pill. Isn't it easier after all to simply take a pill? Surely it is if the alternative is to prepare a meal that meets our needs.

I fear I have bungled my attempt at irony. If there were one task that we should fully invest in, it would be providing for the health and maintenance of our respective machines, the human machine. Though it would be a fool's errand to suggest otherwise, most all of us do exactly that. Time and time again we give short shrift to our physical needs, opting instead to provide for our social desires. It is during those instances when social trumps physical that we turn once more to the pill, the pill of choice in this case being the multivitamin.

A reasonable response you might argue, the idea of supplementing to address a suspected deficiency, but that which makes perfect sense in principle may not be so potent in practice. Here again, I confront one of popular nutrition's hot-button issues. Although the subject of much research and reporting, the role of vitamin supplements in health maintenance and disease prevention remains equivocal. Firmly entrenched in their respective beliefs are the two camps that argue for and against. As is true in most instances involving academic dispute, each side is capable of citing studies that support their positions, and once again, we must arrive at our own truth. In such cases, science does us a disservice. Without proper training (and in many cases even with it), we cannot distinguish between a study that employs good experimental design and one that does not. Consequently we cannot know which results are valid and which are not, which represent good science and which, for want of a better term, is junk science.

In large measure, this inability to distinguish one from the other leaves us vulnerable to assault from either side. In case you have any doubt, know all parties are aware of our gullibility and attack it mercilessly. In the debate about whether or not to supplement, we choose our side and glom onto the science that supports it. For some of us, our conviction becomes so resolute as to approach religious fervor. No matter how compelling the other side's arguments might be, we cannot be dissuaded. Regardless the position you take, you may never know the truth of the matter. I could very easily devote the balance of this book to the citation of research for and against the use of supplements, and in so doing, I would have done nothing to alter any existing beliefs. In fact, my suspicion is, were I to cite research that supports your beliefs, it would go to bolster your position while anything offered contrary to your thinking would be cast aside. An early lesson I learned came from Simon & Garfunkel who sang, "That a man hears what he wants to hear and disregards the rest." From any conversation, we tend to take what we want, which explains why two people can come away from the same conversation with decidedly different interpretations.

On this matter, I will expose my truth not in an effort to sway those who have differing views or to win over those who currently sit on the fence. Rather, it is my purpose to plant my flag, to make my case, to state my beliefs and let them serve as a jumping-off point for future discussions on the subject. Disagree if you must, but hear me out. Our opinions may differ but we are each entitled to them and to their expression.

I believe everything we require is available to us in the form of whole food. By selecting broadly from nature's bounty, we are capable of satisfying our nutrient requirements without need of supplementation. In fact, the very notion that we can do nature one better by packing all the necessary nutrients into a pill half the size of an almond is to me an example of human hubris run amok. I would also argue that the practice of supplementation is based on a logical fallacy. It is assumed by those who supplement that the vitamins contained in their pill of choice are in effect identical to those found in whole food, and as such, the body assimilates them in the same way. So long has this position been held that vitamin manufacturers and distributors no longer need to make the claim. Your work in securing your body's required nutrients begins and ends with taking a pill. An attractive notion to be sure, but is it true?

I will not deny that under certain select conditions some among us would benefit from a multivitamin. That said, it is my general belief that the human body is amazingly adept at extracting from our foods those things we need and very often casting off that which we do not need. The miracle that is the human machine is far too often underappreciated. Complex beyond our understanding, it seems to defy logic that diet and exercise alone are enough to keep our bodies operating at their full potential. Those who have their doubts, look to vitamins as an insurance policy against deficiency, as a quick and easy way to promote good health. In the same way that fuel additives are meant to improve engine performance, vitamins, some believe, improve human performance.

Is it the thought that our diets fail to deliver the necessary nutrients that drive some to supplement or is it the belief that more is better? If it's the former, I would say amend your diet, if it's the latter, amend your thinking. Vitamins are useful in combating deficiencies but offer no additional benefits when taken in doses beyond the recommended daily intake. Yet there are those who promote megadose vitamin therapy for the treatment of select disease states, including cancer. It is not my purpose to argue against such treatment; I will leave that for those better prepared to do so. What I will say is that the idea of it is contrary to what is known about how the body absorbs, stores, and eliminates vitamins.

The dangers tied to excess vitamin intake are both well studied and well understood. This knowledge has not prevented a small number of physicians and others from advancing the megadose theory. What's interesting to me regarding the theory is not so much the theory itself, but rather how it has come in and out of fashion during the past forty plus years.

Dating back to the work of Linus Pauling and others in the early 1970s, megadoses of vitamin C were discussed as a possible cure for cancer and the common cold. Those claims and the research that was said to support them were challenged, and in subsequent clinical trials high dose vitamin C was found to be no more effective than placebo. Despite that finding, miracles connected to mega-dosing the vitamin continue to be reported, if not supported.

If you are among those who practice high dose vitamin therapy, or if you have given thought to it, I encourage you to proceed with caution. As I mentioned, weight loss may not be a science experiment, but many of us treat our bodies as though they are. Experimentation of this type can yield dire consequences. While it would be my recommendation that you not do so, if you are committed to the course, through whatever provocation, I would advise you to solicit the opinion of your physician.

Because not all physicians are well versed in the science of nutrition, a better source for information might be your local registered dietitian. A food and nutrition expert, a dietitian is best positioned to respond to your questions regarding macronutrients (carbohydrates, proteins and fats) and micronutrients (vitamins and minerals). If you had reason to believe or were concerned about the possibility of a vitamin or mineral deficiency, a dietitian could assist you in determining the nature of the deficiency and how best to address it. He or she could provide counsel relative to changes in your diet that would correct the deficiency or, if deemed necessary, recommend an appropriate supplement.

You may wonder why it would be necessary to have someone recommend a supplement when store shelves are full of options. Any one among them should suffice and if not, certainly any of the nationally advertised brands.

You could take as gospel anything that is printed on their labels, or so we may all believe. Confronting this belief is research from Consumerlab.com. A group that has as its mission "to identify the best quality health and nutritional products through independent testing," Consumer Lab did what the government does not, which in the case of this research, meant they tested a select number of supplements for content and quality. Specifically, they purchased forty-two of the leading multivitamin-multimineral supplements sold in North America and put them to the test.

What they discovered was that sixteen of the forty-two failed by some measure to receive their approval. In some cases, the supplement tested was found to have less of a particular nutrient than indicated on the label, while others might have had more. They learned that two of these supplements exceeded the time to breakdown criteria set by the lab. By failing to break apart within the prescribed period (thirty minutes), some portion of the supplement's nutrient profile would not be available for absorption. Of greater concern was the fact that many of the supplements exceeded the upper tolerable intake levels for selected nutrients putting some users, particularly young children, at risk for toxic effects.

Fruit Flavored Supplements

Am I alone in this, or do others find the push to add fruit flavorings to supplements strangely amusing? One product in particular is, to me, especially comical. Sold in the form of gummies, the product is said to deliver four grams of soluble fiber per recommended serving (two gummies). My amusement grows not from the product per se, but rather from the knowledge that one could eat fruit in its natural form and derive as much fiber. In fact, an apple or a pear would provide the same four grams, while a cup of raspberries or blackberries would well exceed that count. Why then would a company not simply recommend people eat fruits and vegetables? A rhetorical question really. We all understand companies exist to make money, and they do not make money when they push products other than those they produce. Not being a shill for those companies, I can comfortably advise you not to purchase these products, and instead find your fiber and other micronutrients conveniently packaged in the form of fruits and vegetables.

I am not an alarmist by nature. For me, the sky is not falling. We cannot live our lives in fear and allow it to dictate our every move. Neither can we be ignorant to what lies ahead. To the extent possible, our decisions, at least the conscious ones, must be reasoned and informed, particularly when those decisions apply to our health. There are a number of unscrupulous individuals on the Internet and elsewhere angling for an opportunity to separate you from your money. In the minds of some, the money they take is in fair compensation for the health enhancing products they promote, whether or not those products do in fact enhance health. For others, their motivation is far more nefarious. Under the guise of competent, caring and credentialed healthcare providers, these characters do, with cruel intent, offer to assist you during your time of need, and help you beat back your infirmity. Oftentimes, they make promises where others did not or could not. Though we must all remain optimistic about our healthcare outcomes, we must also be realistic. Among opinions solicited, if the promise is the outlier, it is fair to consider but not before doing your due diligence. Unless you are well versed in your area of need, do not rely solely upon the explanation given by the practitioner. For all but the most astute, it is easy to become overwhelmed by the proclamations of one capable of talking the talk. As it applies to nutrition, if someone told you that you were deficient in magnesium, zinc and vitamin E, you might be alarmed. You would likely be more alarmed once you knew what role each of these micronutrients play in your body's physiology. Consequently, you could be talked into taking some expensive concoction where no such need existed. Each one of these micronutrients, and every other, is available to you through the foods you eat or the foods you should eat.

Nevertheless, to each of these individuals, our soft and vulnerable underbelly has been exposed. To avoid becoming their victims, we need to be vigilant and ever mindful that they exist not to serve but to fleece. A common practice for those who do is to identify a particular micronutrient or phytochemical that either has been in the news or has been the topic of public discourse. They then gin up the significance of the nutrient, perhaps exaggerating its effects or fabricating them outright. Either way, their claims are usually gross misrepresentations of the truth, if not bald-faced lies. From these distortions, they fear no consequences, because for every person who sees through their ruse there are many more who will fall victim to it. So they create a new product featuring the nutrient, or simply add it to an existing product and then sit back and wait for the money to roll in.

Three examples that come immediately to mind are those of beta-carotene, lutein, and lycopene. Antioxidants all, each of these phytonutrients have found their way onto the labels of virtually every multivitamin sold in the United States. If their presence in the multi's fails to meet your need, each is also available as a stand-alone supplement. But what truly is your need and does supplementing achieve it?

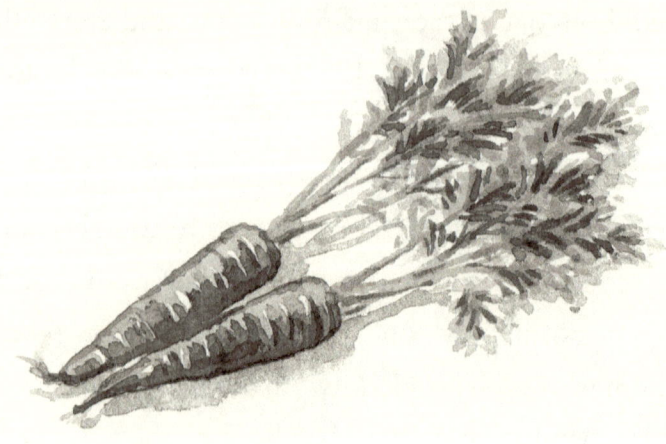

For none of the three is a specific daily intake recommended; however, with regard to beta-carotene one website advises those who visit to consume twenty-five thousand IU daily. Because, they claim, it would be difficult to accomplish through diet alone they recommend that one supplement. Offered as an inducement for doing so is the following list of health benefits for beta-carotene supplements.

- Provides relief from carpal tunnel and repetitive stress injuries
- Relieves symptoms of osteoarthritis and rheumatoid arthritis
- Protects against UV radiation from the sun
- Prevents diabetes, relieves symptoms of diabetes
- Prevents cataracts and macular degeneration
- Enhances the function of the immune system
- Prevents many types of cancer

- Increases strength and endurance
- Improves prostate function
- Improves recovery time from exercise
- Reduces pain and inflammation
- Promotes healthy eyesight
- Promotes cardiovascular health
- Relieves respiratory system problems
- Beneficial for male and female fertility

It goes on to list the health conditions for which beta-carotene supplements are recommended, although it fails to indicate whom it is that makes these recommendations. The conditions include:

- AIDS
- Asthma
- Bronchitis and emphysema
- Cataracts
- Cervical and prostate cancer
- Lung cancer
- Chlamydial infection
- Diabetes
- Eczema and psoriasis
- Heart disease
- Male and female infertility
- Osteoarthritis

- Photosensitivity
- Pneumonia
- Rheumatoid arthritis
- Skin cancer
- Vaginal candidiasis
- Macular degeneration

All right already, sign me up! One would have to admit that these are some powerful, and, to some, persuasive claims. Even if you were dubious about the claims, you might be tempted to give it a go. A relatively small cost, you might reason, with the prospect, no matter how slight, of significant returns in terms of your health. And in that moment of weakness, of uncertainty, you fall into their snare.

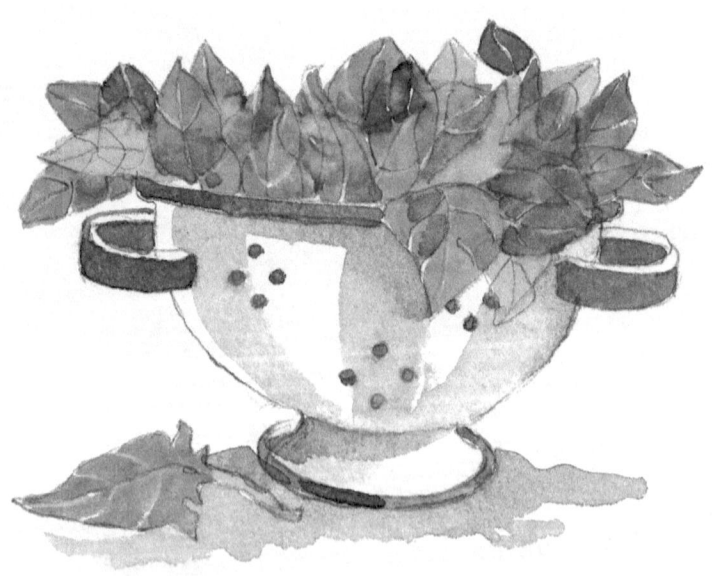

With regard to lutein and lycopene, similar snares have been set. According to a study commissioned by the Dietary Supplement Education Alliance (DSEA), not, by the way, what I would consider an unbiased source, taking 6-10 milligrams of lutein daily could spare 190,000 individuals the need to access care from nursing facilities secondary to macular degeneration. As a consequence, it was estimated that $3.6 billion could be saved over a five-year period. Here they appeal not only to our fear of dependence but also to fear of financial ruin.

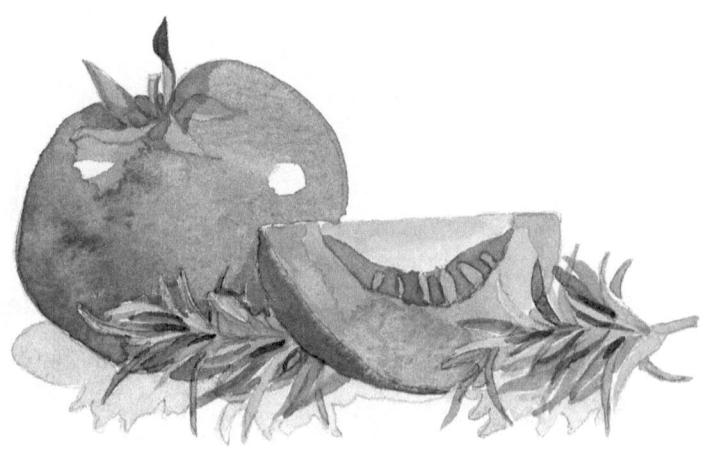

Equally outlandish are claims regarding lycopene. Found commonly in tomatoes and tomato-based preparations, lycopene has been associated with a number of positive health outcomes including the reduction of LDL cholesterol and a somewhat more speculative benefit to prostate health. Those who advocate that you supplement lycopene have extrapolated these findings to include a variety of other conditions, among which are lung, breast, ovarian, pancreatic, skin, and stomach cancer. Once again, if the prospect of developing one of these cancers causes you to live your life in fear, these claims could easily persuade you to add lycopene to your growing list of supplements. After all, what is the price for peace of mind? Whatever the price, the peace of mind you buy with lycopene supplements, or supplements in general, particularly as it applies to disease prevention, is at best supposed and not established as real or true.

Supporting this thinking is research published in the *British Medical Journal* (BMJ 2013; 346:f10). Authors of the referenced study examined fifty trials involving nearly three hundred thousand participants. Based upon their analysis of those trials the authors concluded, "There is no evidence to support the use of vitamin and antioxidant supplements for prevention of cardiovascular diseases."

Powerful as this research may be, I do not expect it to close the book on the subject of vitamins and their role in disease prevention. Those with conflicting opinions can, have, and will likely continue to introduce evidence of their own in an effort to consolidate public opinion in favor of supplementation. While it continues to be my position that all the nutrients and micronutrients we require are available to us in sufficient quantity through the foods we eat, I will make no further attempt to win you over. If you are among those who supplement and derive some comfort from doing so, carry on. If you buy into the adage that 10 percent of something is better than 100 percent of nothing, then I will not stand in your way. Like all decisions related to your health, they are yours to make. You must decide for yourself if there is truth in the claims offered by the vitamin industry. As you attempt to make sense of the arguments for and against, please consider that trite expression: if a thing sounds too good to be true, it probably is. Concerning the claimed benefits of the phytonutrients mentioned above, I can think of nothing that sounds better. I'll leave it to your own good judgment to decide if the claims are too good.

Chapter 10

What's on the Menu?

It was never on my bucket list, but when the opportunity presented to attend the Houston Rodeo, I jumped at it. It is reputed to be the world's largest entertainment and livestock exhibition, and while I had no particular interest in livestock or the wrestling and roping thereof, it was the event in its entirety that attracted me. I admit, I was a stranger to the world of rodeo, but it was as a stranger that my curiosity was piqued. During the course of my life, I have attempted to expose myself to as many unique experiences as possible, if for no other reason but to broaden my horizon. To say that the Houston Rodeo was for me unique would be a gross mischaracterization of the event.

I will remember much about the day I spent there, but it is sad, I think, that my strongest memory will be of the food items made available for purchase. In an article on the subject, the Houston Fox affiliate wrote, "One of the biggest attractions at the annual Houston Livestock Show and Rodeo is the food. Fried, sugared, roasted, you name it, they got it." The article goes on to address the Gold Buckle Foodie Awards presented to food vendors in eight distinct categories including best food-on-a-stick, best classic fair food, best fried food, and best dessert, among others. In a thinly veiled attempt to move as much food as possible, the rodeo brain trust devised the I Ate All 8 Challenge. Interested rodeo-goers are given a punch card listing all eight first-place winners. Their mission, contrary to the title of the contest, is to eat five of the eight award winning entries. Once they have done so they are instructed to deliver their cards to the show's social station. The first fifty who do so receive a Houston Livestock Show and Rodeo cookbook. My first thought was that it's not bad enough that you're made to eat five fat-laden foods, but you must also do it for time or you risk not receiving your cookbook. It seemed to me that a more appropriate prize, given the demands of the contest, would have been a free angioplasty.

I won't get into the rodeo's role in promoting unhealthy eating practices, where nutrition is concerned the rodeo should not be confused with the Mayo Clinic. Beyond that,

I feel the majority of folks attending this event go at least in part with the expectation of finding such delicacies. As one sign indicated, "It's the Rodeo, to Hell with the Diet". The question is, do these foods fit, and if so, where and or how, within a healthy diet, let alone one that has as its purpose to bring about weight loss?

I think it is appropriate at this point that we stop for a moment, take a deep breath, and reflect on the notion that we each have a finite amount of time on this planet. Remembering my admonition from chapter 1 that none of us gets out of this alive, we do have choices to make about the lives we lead. If it is our choice to live our lives overweight, we are free to do so. If, on the other hand, we choose to lead a life free from the encumbrance of excess weight, then that too is our right. However, rights come with responsibilities and the responsibility we accept when we agree to live our lives thus is to keep our overindulgences in check. With that as a responsibility, partaking in deep-fried Oreos (yes, they too were on sale at the rodeo) would be an exceptionally rare treat.

Thinking of such foods as a desirable treat, or worse yet, as a staple within your diet speaks to a fundamental psychological difference between the overweight and those who are not. Although certainly not true in every case, those who are at or near normal weight tend to view items such as the deep-fried Oreo as at best a perverse curiosity.

To the extent that they're given thought to at all, Oreos in general, never mind those that are deep-fried, are not mourned when unavailable as a snack. The overweight, if you'll allow me another broad-brush characterization, might be more likely to see the Oreo, and perhaps particularly the deep-fried version as a tempting taste treat. Within the context of the rodeo they might be hard-pressed to take a pass, reasoning, "Where else but here?"

It is in that anxiety of to pass or not to pass where a chief distinction lies; an anxiety that I contend is born out of our emotional attachment to food. I believe the most difficult task faced by all who struggle with their weight comes not from removing foods from their diet, but rather from removing the emotional attachments they have for those foods. How often have you heard a friend or family member use the word *love* to describe their feelings for a particular food item? We all understand the word love. We use it to describe intense feelings of affection. Oftentimes we apply it in a romantic or sexual sense. For those who use the word love to give meaning to the depth of emotion they feel for their favorite foods, I do not believe that it is misapplied. I do not exaggerate when I say I have heard people describe their response to certain foods in a manner that stops just short of a shuddering orgasm. It is interesting to me that our feelings for a spouse or loved one may change overtime but our feelings for food remain constant. In fact, if our rates of divorce and obesity are any indication it may be easier to end a marriage than to end our emotional bond with food.

Conversely, when conversations turn toward those food items we find especially objectionable, the word *hate* is often employed. Regrettably the word seems to be reserved for vegetables such as broccoli, brussels sprouts, in fact, sprouts of any kind, cauliflower and the like. Up to this point in my life, I have yet to hear the word *hate* used by anyone as they describe their feelings for bacon. Even in my own case, as someone who has not eaten bacon in many years, I could not correctly say that I hate bacon, I simply choose not to include it in my diet. The subject of multiple "Fests" around the country each year, bacon is America's cured meat of choice; sad to imagine that we have one.

I mention these powerful words of emotion in context to our relationship with food as a means of underscoring the difficult task we have at hand. I don't need to tell you that love and hate are our most emotionally charged words. Using either word to describe your feelings for another person will have a significant influence on that relationship going forward. Using the same words to describe your feelings for food does nothing to change your feelings; it simply puts an exclamation point on them and leads us back to the challenges we confront in our efforts to break the stranglehold that food has in our lives.

In their book entitled *Super Foods Rx - Fourteen Foods That Will Change Your Life* authors Steven Pratt and Kathy Matthews offer compelling testimony for the health giving, life-altering effects of a select list of foods that include beans, blueberries, broccoli, oats, oranges, pumpkin, wild salmon, soy, spinach, tea, tomatoes, turkey (specifically skinless breast), walnuts, and yogurt. Before making their case for each, they appeal to their readers to give careful thought to their food choices. They argue that by choosing their book, the reader has come to a critical "fork in the road" where their health is concerned. Go one way, they claim, and you'll spend your retirement washing down prescription medications while seated in front of the television. Choose the other path, and rather than retiring into quiet desperation, your golden years will be filled with fun and frolic - hyperbole at its finest!

I offer this reference in part because I, like Pratt and Matthews, believe that with respect to our food we can make better choices. Excellent though I think their choices are, I do believe that the term *super food* might itself be hyperbolic. Super or not their fourteen foods do speak to the concept of nutrient density that I have attempted to shine a light on in previous chapters. All of the foods they highlight are nutrient density incarnate, tangible examples of foods that are veritable warehouses of the nutrients we require to survive and thrive.

Still, while I support their founding principle that we can and must endeavor to make wiser food choices, we part company when they tacitly suggest that one only needs to *choose* as though doing so were as simple as getting out of bed in the morning. In this book, I have droned on and on about choice. Choosing one thing over another may be a simple matter up until the time that emotion becomes involved. Without having to be told, we each know that where nutrition is concerned, a cup of blueberries is far preferable to a cup of French fries. Unfortunately, for those who *love* French fries that knowledge does nothing to ease the decision or alter the choice.

Yes, relative to our diet, each day we are presented with choices. Making decisions based on the choices offered should not be seen as equivalent to choosing which pair of socks to put on in the morning. To those who would have you believe otherwise, I would say it is a difficult matter to undo a pattern of behavior established during the course of one's lifetime. For those of you who do grapple with your food choices, good and bad, know that positive change is possible. Difficult though it may be to achieve, it can be done, and for the sake of your health in the long-term, must be done.

When faced with a particularly difficult dilemma, some among us seek divine intervention. Others hope for a bit of magic. If the dilemma you face is your inability to put aside your lustful feelings for the foods that wield power in your life, know there are no elixirs to take that would remove the mouth-watering flavor from a bacon cheeseburger. There are no spells that could be cast that would leave one feeling no less emotionally satisfied following a large salad than they would be after a fried chicken dinner. Such sorcery simply does not exist. Which is not to say that success can't be yours. Success is possible if only through more earthly means. Rather than employing witchcraft, the change in behavior we seek will instead be brought about through the introduction of reinforcing stimulus. With weight loss as the goal, if patterning the appropriate behaviors in terms of exercise and food consumption yields the desired result (namely decreased weight), it will increase the likelihood that those behaviors will be continued. No, as I have said before we do not need to eliminate the more calorie-dense items from your diet; we simply need to put them in proper proportion so that they represent a relatively small percentage of your total intake.

Your feelings for bacon cheeseburgers and fried chicken may never change. If they are among the foods you find most satisfying, or otherwise have a strong connection to, it will be nigh impossible to alter your perceptions. Instead, it would be my aim to help you see that they are contrary to your purposes of achieving and sustaining a healthy weight. I have argued that those purposes can be achieved even in the presence of these foods; however, some will find it exceedingly difficult to do so. It is in some ways analogous to a failed relationship in that while you may attempt to remain friends following the end of a romantic relationship, not all will be successful, for some, it will be necessary to make a clean break. I can't know who among you will be able to *end* your "romantic" relationship with the calorie dense foods that have contributed to the challenges you presently face and instead establish a new connection, wherein they can continue to be a part of your life but in a much-diminished way. The amorous feelings you harbor for such foods may make maintaining a casual relationship unthinkable. As it is my general belief that weight loss programs fail in part because they ask too much of the dieter; I have attempted to keep the door to the inclusion of all foods open. You alone must decide for yourself whether that door can remain open or if it should be barred shut to exclude foods with which you have had, and would expect to continue to have, an unhealthy bond.

If you have already begun to apply some of the principles discussed in previous chapters, you may know without need of much introspection whether, or to what degree, your *love* foods can be featured in your diet. Regardless of your thinking on that subject, it has been my purpose to make weight loss a less punitive process. Under the best of circumstances, many of us battle with body image issues and low self-esteem, adding unwanted weight to the equation can only serve to make matters worse. Rather than heaping on additional bitter feelings, I had hoped to ease you into weight loss by making subtle changes to your eating behaviors. Better, I believe to let time be an ally. If your patience allows, manage your weight loss to keep it from managing you.

A critical step in this process, and one that was first discussed in chapter 2, requires you to control your portions. In that chapter, I suggested you reveal more of your plate by making it less fully occupied with food. If you have implemented that step, yet still struggle with portion size, consider what I would expect you'd find to be the an unusual recommendation - frozen food. Not just any frozen food, but rather those selections intended as healthy alternatives to home cooking. I offer this suggestion being fully aware of the limitations and complications associated with these foods. Many frozen meals contain disproportionately high percentages of sodium and fat. The worst offenders offer unhealthy quantities of saturated fat and trans fat. So with this recommendation comes the important proviso that you read the label. Do not assume that those meals marketed as being lean options deliver on their promise. In addition to the obvious concern about calories, be mindful of the meal's saturated fat, cholesterol and sodium content and endeavor to keep them at or preferably below, 10 percent of the recommended daily values. Please know the manufacturer did not place the label there thinking it would be a good idea. Instead, our government mandated its inclusion believing that the information it provides would allow consumers to make more informed decisions regarding their food choices.

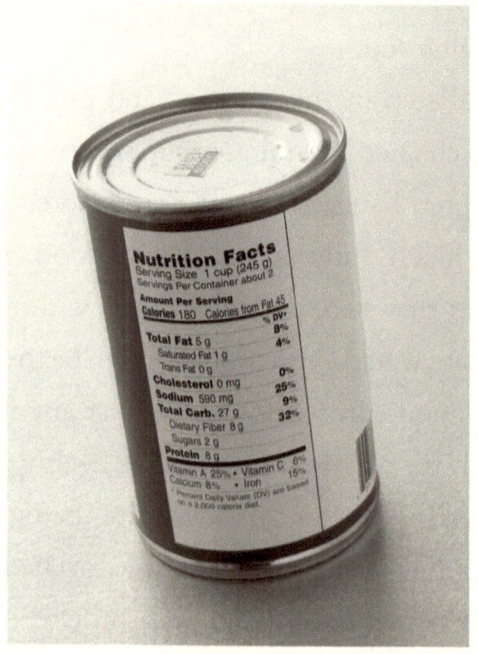

Those of you who have tried frozen meals know that adhering to the above referenced criteria eliminates a great many options straightaway. However, in the ongoing effort to control our energy intake, we need to get a clearer picture of what a serving of food should look like. Despite their other limitations, I believe these meals when selected according to the listed criteria achieve that aim.

For those of you who have embarked on this weight loss quest alone, the appropriately selected frozen meal has the added benefit of not leaving any leftovers behind. In and of themselves, leftovers are not necessarily a bad thing. The more creative among us can craft the leavings from one meal into a seemingly unrelated new meal. However, for those who struggle to lose weight, any uneaten portion of a meal all too frequently becomes a portion of the same meal. It's just a couple or a few bites we reason; there's no point dirtying a container to store it away for the night, so I'll just finish it off. And we do, not because we're still hungry but because the food is there. These meals subtract out that temptation, contained within each box is exactly one meal. From having read the nutrition label, you know the precise calorie count without need for weighing or measuring.

While I would certainly prefer that our meals be fresh out of the a garden or at the very least fresh out of the a produce section, I do realize that the frenetic pace with which we lead our lives makes such preparations at times impossible. On those occasions when life requires you to take your meals at a fast jog, the carefully selected frozen meal is a viable option. On this point, I do not doubt that others will disagree. Some among them are certain to burn me in effigy for daring to make such a suggestion. I make it knowing that it might not be the best choice, but rather a convenient one that offers some unique advantages to those who are attempting to exercise control over their energy intake.

Should you decide to avail yourself of one of these meals, try to choose one that brings some color to your plate. To remove the mystery from that prior sentence, by color, I mean a fruit or vegetable. In the event one is not included, be certain to amend the meal with a small salad or a serving or two of fruit.

Dependent upon your perspective, it is either a blessing or a curse that allows us to eat so freely from fruits and vegetables. They represent the one category of food that I encourage people to select from liberally. Within their variety it is possible to find much of what our bodies require. Add in some whole grain breads, rice, and pasta, a selection of nuts and beans, a few servings of reduced fat or fat free dairy products, accent with fish and meat, and you have what should constitute the majority of your daily food intake.

I have not included meat and dairy to rankle the more militant vegans among us. For what it's worth, I have respect for those who have made the choice to live their lives in the absence of animal products. Yet in the final analysis, it is a choice, and they alone are bound to it. Others who do not wish to be so constrained should feel free to include meat, fish, poultry and dairy in their diets.

With regard to dairy in particular, the radical nutritionists would have you believe that we humans should not drink milk. Arguing that we are the only animal who drinks the milk of another species, they claim this practice demonstrates a lack of compassion for cows and it is otherwise unhealthy for a whole host of reasons. On the point of our exploitation of cows, I simply can't get comfortable with the idea that because other species don't drink cow's milk neither should we. I believe that if those other species were able to extract milk from a cow, they would happily drink it; cats certainly don't hesitate when we set a bowl down in front of them. As to the supposed health effects of milk, I would say we're each entitled to our own truth but not our own facts. Facts are pieces of information that serve to establish a thing as being certain or true. You'll hear the word thrown around frequently, and in almost every case, it is misemployed. A thing is not a fact simply because it is said to be so, and it does not gain in strength by being stated more fervently or more loudly. Let us not confuse what we believe to be true with what is known to be true.

What is known to be true about our food choices is that they are ours to make. While I have attempted to highlight those selections I believe are most helpful to you as you search for answers to your weight loss dilemma, I will not pretend that they serve everyone equally well. We are all unique individuals with needs, wants, and desires peculiar to us alone. To prescribe a program with the expectation that it would or could be applied uniformly across generations, ethnic groups, cultures, and socioeconomic standings is foolhardy. What I have offered are recommendations; they have not been chiseled in stone and carried down from the mountaintop. In them, it is my sincere hope that you will find useful information that you can call upon when faced with the sometimes-difficult decisions that grow out of your determination to lose weight.

Chapter 11

Dining Out

Why is it that restaurants continue to offer dishes that are excessively high in their calorie content? Because they sell! On this point, let's not blame the restaurants for providing for the wants of their clientele. Restaurants, regardless of their stripe, are doing nothing more than catering to the whims and wishes of those they serve. Holding them out as villains in our ongoing issues with weight is, I think, unfair. In my mind, it is equivalent to condemning the media for sensationalizing death, destruction and mayhem. They do so for the same reason that restaurants sell fatty foods - because it pays the bills.

Rest assured that if restaurants were inundated with requests for low-calorie dishes, they would fall all over themselves to make those dishes available to their diners. As is true with most businesses, it is not their ideology, but rather the all-consuming pursuit of the dollar bill that guides their practices.

It is also true that actions speak louder than words. While there are voices being heard that have called for these changes, those changes that have been instituted appear to have had little influence on the purchasing habits of their base patrons. As a result, the low-calorie options have, in the main, gained little traction. It seems the richer menu items continue to be those that most folks gravitate toward.

In an effort to address concerns about our rising girth and what that portends for our society as a whole, legislation was passed (The Patient Protection and Affordable Care Act of 2010), which, among others things, is intended to assist diners in making better choices for the food they eat away from home. Hotly debated for reasons other than those mentioned here, the act requires that restaurants post the number of calories for each of their menu items. By so posting the act seeks to reverse our current trend through the power of information.

Like the 1990 Nutrition Labeling and Education Act before it, the 2010 legislation aims to provide consumers with the tools needed to select those foods that provide the best nutrition, or at the very least, allows them to distinguish between the foods that do and those that do not. Although not fully implemented at the time of this writing, a small number of states and local jurisdictions have already jumped onboard. However, in those regions where the legislation has been implemented, is it achieving the desired result? At this point, the answer remains very much in doubt. While some studies of menu labeling have demonstrated what might be referred to as a modest reduction in the number of calories purchased (as compared with the pre-implementation rate), others show no change at all.

It may be sometime before we can draw any definitive conclusions regarding the efficacy of menu labeling laws, but at this point, I think it is fair to say the results have been underwhelming. Without knowing the full intent of those who created this legislation, I would guess they had hoped restaurant goers would be swayed by the calorie cost when making their selections. With a burger on their minds, would they choose a wrap when confronted with the calorie differential? Considering the early returns, it would appear the answer to this question is no. To the extent that they acknowledge the information at all, it seems that most folks have chosen to simply carry on living their lives. Maybe it's because they don't appreciate the significance of those numbers, or they have no idea what their daily caloric allotment should be, or maybe they believe that life is too short to be spent worrying about calories.

On their point that life is too short, I agree; it is too short to be impeded by unwanted weight, it is too short to be spent wondering how it might be different minus the stored fat, and it is too short to live with the fear of chronic disease and the limitations it imposes. It goes back to lifestyle choices; how we choose to live the life we've been given. It is ours to do with as we please, if there are any aspects within our lives that leave us unfulfilled, we can continue to gnash our teeth or we can take steps to change our course. As it pertains to our weight either we can continue to add to it, or we can do the things to help us subtract from it.

Dependent upon your political leanings, you may look at menu labeling as an unnecessary governmental intrusion into existing business practices, or you may think of it as a helping hand in our collective effort to reign in obesity. While I must say I applaud the effort, I have my doubts about its ultimate affect. Yes, people should choose foods throughout the course of their day that they enjoy, but also fit within their daily calorie allotment. For those who have that as their goal, providing calorie data will be useful. For those who can't be bothered, it is an exercise in futility.

I recall a dinner out in Charleston, South Carolina a few years back. After having reviewed the menu, the other members of my party and I began to make our selections. One in the party, curious about a beef dish wrapped in bacon, asked the server if he thought that particular choice was a good one. Apparently caught off guard by the question, the server looked at him as though he had just arrived here from another planet. "Of course it's good", he said, "It has bacon wrapped around it". How is one to argue with that kind of logic?

If I had had any interest in the dish, the question I would have asked is, how many calories and grams of saturated fat does it contain? However, in the case of my friend, who ultimately ordered the item, his only concern was whether he would enjoy it. On that account, he was not disappointed, but he, and in fact we all, must consider the consequences of our food choices wherever we take our meals. It is for this reason that menu labeling has value. If you truly crave a burger then perhaps the 240-calorie variety will be no less successful at satisfying that urge than the one thousand plus calorie option would be.

The assistance offered through the discussed legislation is as much as we can hope for, and even in its case, opposition was fierce. The restaurant industry claimed that the act would place undue burden on small business owners who would be made to bear the costs associated with the implementation, execution, and additional employee training needed to comply with the act. But comply they must. Don't imagine for one minute that those who fall under the scope of the act have complied, or ultimately will, out of some sense of social conscience. In what is an admittedly warped view of American business, I believe there are only two explanations for why they do what they do – first because they're paid to, and second because they're made to.

When made to, resistance always precedes acquiescence. In the case of the act, the restaurant industry, like a petulant child, offers up all the reasons why they shouldn't do what they're being made to do. One of the reasons the industry offered for not being saddled with this new legislation was their belief that the act will bear no fruit when it comes to curbing obesity. This is the same position that the beverage industry took when Mayor Bloomberg attempted to regulate the size of soft drinks in New York City. If either industry had any inclination to act on behalf of the public good, they might say, "Sure, let's give this a try". Instead, they hide behind the Constitution suggesting the right to hold and bear forty-eight ounce Cokes or an eighteen-hundred-calorie hamburger is an inalienable right. Whether inalienable or not, I believe if a person wants to buy a bucket of Coke and a side of beef on a bun they should be free to do so, provided that both are available for purchase. Similarly, a restaurant should be free to sell those items if they so choose. However, I would not expect to hear an objection from either party when it comes to the posting of nutrition information. I do believe that withholding that information is taking the thought of buyer beware too far. We cannot divine the number of calories contained in meals we take while away from home. In addition, it is not for the restaurant industry to decide whether or not that is information that we need to know. If managing our calories is an important component of managing our weight, which I contend, it is, then this is information that needs to be made readily available. Let us the buyers decide whether, or to what degree, we utilize the information. While it's my preference that we not consume ourselves with the numbers, at the very least we must be cognizant of them. Once we've established a foundation of information regarding the calorie content of a variety of foods, we can use that knowledge to arrive at a rough estimate of the calorie content of similar or related foods.

Knowing our daily calorie allotment and the approximate calorie content of the foods we eat will assist us in maintaining our existing weight or subtracting from it. However, even when in possession of this information, we must be careful to mind the temptations that life throws in our paths. It is for this reason that I advise those who are intent on losing weight, to avoid family style and buffet restaurants. While I'm certain the owners of these establishments would object to being singled out, after all temptation surrounds us, my particular objection to the aforementioned restaurants relates to the quantity of food served. In the case of the family style restaurants, for those unfamiliar, items ordered are typically served on platters allowing diners to load their plates according to their own desires. Dependent upon the size of the party and the number of items ordered, this could become a prescription for overeating, especially if some quantity of food hasn't been claimed at the end of the meal. Like leftovers at home, the last vestiges of the meal are sure to find their way on to someone's plate.

Worse still, in my mind, are the buffet restaurants. For a flat fee patrons can return to the trough as often as they wish, eating until it is physically impossible to continue. The only thing standing between them and doing so is the ability to recognize when enough is enough. For some among us, purchasing calories is no different from purchasing any other item or service; we must get as much as possible of it, whatever *it* happens to be. When weight loss is the objective, this is fatal thinking. Rather than focusing on the number of calories your money buys, instead pay attention to the composition and quality of your calories.

For those on a tight budget, this can become especially problematic. Widely reported and undisputed is the fact that a person's income bears heavily in his or her food choices. When cost becomes a factor, those of limited means are more likely to opt for less healthy options, whether eating at home or dining out. All of that said, a person can, regardless of their financial circumstances, make better choices. Without intending to minimize the difficulty associated with making those choices when one is financially disadvantaged, it is, nevertheless, possible to avoid the calorie-dense and nutrient-deprived alternatives. Even among restaurants in the quick-service category, healthy choices are experiencing an uptick in sales. While burgers, fries and pizza continue to be the sales leaders, salads, fruits and leaner sandwich options are making headway.

Whatever your financial circumstance, if weight loss is your goal, know that it is achievable. Whether rich, poor, or something in between, the prescription for its accomplishment is exactly the same - eat less and move more. On the eating side of the equation, when dining out in those restaurants that provide calorie information, use it to assist with your selections. In those restaurants that do not offer the data don't hesitate to ask it of your server. Whether posted or not, most restaurants, at least those with multiple locations, (i.e. chain restaurants), have the information and can provide it to you upon request. As mentioned previously, while we don't want to obsess about the numbers, we do want to be mindful of them. It is better, I think, to be aware of them before eating than surprised by them after.

Family Restaurant Fatties			
Restaurant	Menu Item	Calories	Saturated Fats (grams)
P.F. Chang's China Bistro	Pork Fried Rice	1370	8
California Pizza Kitchen	Pesto Cream Penne with Chicken and Shrimp	1620	58
Chili's Bar & Grill	Honey Chipotle Chicken Crispers with Ranch	1660	13
Applebee's Neighborhood Grill	New England Fish and Chips	1690	22
Macaroni Grill	Chianti Barbeque Steak	1920	42
The Old Spaghetti Factory	Hearty Mizithra and Brown Butter	1990	74
The Cheesecake Factory	Bistro Shrimp Pasta	2290	73
Maggiano's Little Italy	Veal Porterhouse	2400	52
Claim Jumper	Ore Cart	2724	72

Table assembled using information collected from the respective restaurant's websites

Chapter 12

A Place to Keep Our Stuff

Stacked up against the span of time that we, or those like us, have roamed the planet, our ability to effectively preserve and store food has been a relatively recent phenomenon. While it is true that our distant ancestors had begun smoking and curing meat (as a means of preserving it for later consumption) many centuries ago, it was not until the latter nineteenth century, a veritable blink of the eye, that refrigeration first became available to the American consumer. Even then it was not widely employed until the 1940s.

Developing along or about the same timeline was the commercial process for canning food. Not made broadly available until the 1880s, canned foods gained in popularity in the 1930s and 1940s, falling off secondary to rationing in the middle forties, and then regaining vigor in the latter forties and beyond. Today we find canned foods in varying quantities in homes across America and around the world.

Hunters and gatherers no more, we have adapted our lifestyles and our kitchens to accommodate these conveniences. A home built today that does not feature a walk-in pantry or a refrigerator larger than some Parisian apartments would cause a number of prospective buyers to walk away in disgust. Storage, it seems, is a problem for us all, and increasingly so within our kitchens.

The late comedian George Carlin referred to our homes as the place where we keep our "stuff", as a "pile of stuff with a lid on it". If you accept that as true, it is also true that our kitchens are the places within our homes where we pile our food. Walk into the average American kitchen and you are likely to find cupboards brimming and refrigerators engorged with food of every description; from processed and prepackaged to fresh from the farm, we Americans can't bear the idea of being more than a few feet away from something to eat.

Of course, it is reasonable and appropriate to have some quantity of food on hand in anticipation of meals to come. After all, running to the store every day to purchase supplies for that day's meals would be a nuisance and a bother, right? For we Americans the answer would appear to be yes, but among those countries in which people are more likely to shop multiple times during the week, if not daily, rates of obesity are significantly lower.

The inference is obvious although not totally intended – people who store less food tend to eat less food. That said it would be wrong to suggest that the degree to which we Americans store food is the only difference between people of other cultures and ourselves. There are many fine, and some gross, distinctions between how others and we prepare, consume, and relate to food. It is, I think, the sum total of these distinctions and not simply that we store a disproportionately large quantity of food that sets us apart from others and makes us more likely to fall into the trap that is obesity.

Still, the act of storing food is not as innocent as it otherwise might appear. Stored food ultimately becomes consumed food and sometimes sooner than intended. I don't think anyone would argue that the more easily one is able to access food the more likely he or she is to eat it, and oftentimes for reasons other than to satisfy hunger.

We have all, at one time or another, caught ourselves staring blankly into our refrigerators and cupboards. Not necessarily motivated by hunger but just because we happened to be passing through the kitchen or wandered in during a lull in our TV programming. At times such as these, we are vulnerable to eating for the sake of eating. In these cases, eating becomes something to do; it is a means of occupying our idle moments, a way in which we can pass time. This, I contend, is an especially dangerous practice and one I'm afraid is unique to we Americans.

This is not directly tied to our TV viewing habits, as other nations have caught up to us in terms of hours spent in front of the tube, but rather related to our enduring oral fixation. I personally wonder how it's possible to free up a hand long enough to convey a food item to our mouths when our hands are otherwise occupied manipulating our tablets and smart phones, a practice in which nearly 90 percent of us engage while watching television. Apparently, these second screen interactions have done little to deter us from satisfying our overriding obsession with food, which brings me back to the pursuit of squirreling food away. As mentioned, we do so at rates far beyond that of other countries. In part, it is a function of the space we have to fill; if there is room in our cupboards and refrigerators we tend to fill them. Unlike Old Mother Hubbard from the English nursery rhyme of the same name, few of us are in danger of discovering our cupboards to be bare.

However, I believe, there is more at work here than a well thought out plan of emergency preparedness. We are not storing food away in anticipation of some natural disaster. The food we store now will not be around for any such calamity. It is food that is meant to be eaten, some as part of our meals, and some specifically for the purposes of between meal snacking. In this latter role, we must take care to ensure that the available selections are both nutritious and spare in terms of their calorie content. If we fail in this effort, we increase the likelihood that we will end our day with a calorie surplus.

The message here is to be wary when stocking your food storage areas. Whether you're doing so for yourself or for your family, limit or eliminate those foods that pass along calories and little else. Avoid foods packed in bags, sleeves, cartons, and the like, which make it entirely too easy to exceed a single serving. And choose fruits and vegetables over processed and packaged items. This one action will help to control your calorie intake by preferentially selecting items that are naturally lower in their per serving calorie count.

Regardless an item's calorie count, it's important to be mindful of why you're eating what you're eating. As you strive to make changes to your weight, know there is precious little margin for error in your daily-caloric consumption. Make any such errors on the side of eating too little rather than too much. If the thought of doing so leaves you filled with anxiety, worry not. Learning to live with less than you want may be a problem, but getting by with less than you expect you need is not. Dependent upon the quantity of fat you have stored and your goals related to doing away with that fat, it might be necessary to remain in calorie deficit for some time to come, but in the end the result will have been worth the effort.

Chapter 13

⌒⁓

Creating Your Masterpiece

Perhaps best known as the artist who created the *Mona Lisa*, Leonardo da Vinci was one of mankind's greatest thinkers. His work became the harbinger for many inventions that would not see the light of day until modern times. A man of apparently limitless interest and intellect Leonardo da Vinci's surviving work demonstrates a keen understanding of a great many subjects not the least of which was human anatomy. Although doodles by comparison to his master work, he sketched numerous illustrations depicting various aspects of our surface and deep anatomy. Masterful in their own right, these drawings afford us the opportunity to inspect those structures that lie beneath in their most intricate detail.

Focusing not on anatomy per se but rather on human proportions, is Leonardo da Vinci's work entitled the *Vitruvian Man*. Through it, da Vinci explores the balance and symmetry inherent in human beings. Whether the subject portrayed in the piece is typical of fifteenth-century man I can't know, but I would be unchallenged if I were to assert that he is not typical of twenty-first-century man. Da Vinci's model was lithe and well muscled and as such would be representative of only a small percentage of today's man. Were a similar project commissioned today, with the objective of displaying not the ideal but rather the typical man, the finished product would be vastly different. The modern day model would be decidedly doughier, not obese necessarily, but certainly overfat.

If you meet this description and aspire to become a modern day *Vitruvian Man* (or woman), you will most likely not get there by following the course thus far outlined in this book. My objective has been to put you on a path to achievable and sustainable weight loss, to help you establish or reestablish a more viable relationship with the food you eat, and to welcome activity into your life. If by following my recommendations you have begun to appreciate some positive change in your weight and have been spurred on to confront still greater challenges, know that with sustained effort and commitment all things are possible.

Dependent upon your specific goals, the activities we spoke of in previous chapters may not be of sufficient intensity or duration to bring about the changes you seek. While I continue to support walking as a weight loss activity, if it, in combination with calorie restriction has begun to pare off the pounds, it may be possible to introduce jogging to your program. I use the word *may* because the transition from walking to jogging increases the stresses applied to the weight-bearing joints (hips, knees, ankles and feet). To minimize the risk of injury to these structures, it is in my mind, preferable to reduce the load they are asked to bear to a weight below their tolerable limit. Because that weight varies, dependent upon your unique bony anatomy, it is advisable for you to seek the counsel of your physician before embarking on a jogging program. With that said, given an equal investment in terms of time, jogging has a higher calorie cost than does walking. If you implemented no further changes to your program, jogging alone would accelerate your weight loss.

Whether jogging now or just giving thought to the possibility it could represent a sea change in your attitude toward exercise. Previously, I spoke of successful exercise experiences early inviting opportunities to explore exercise of greater demand later, and progressing from walking to jogging serves as an excellent example. The very idea of it may have at one point caused you to think, "Who me?

Hell, no!" However, if you discovered that walking along with modifications to your diet yielded positive change, you might begin to wonder just how much more you can achieve. On that point, I will set no bounds. Your return is in direct proportion to the size of your investment. Ask more of yourself physically, and for every minute of added effort, you will be repaid with increased calories burned.

You say that you have not come to that point where you're able to take on the challenge of jogging. Don't let that deter you; weight loss is a stepwise progression. If walking has served you well, continue walking, but in the interest of adding to the intensity, quicken your pace. Another option to consider would be to intersperse your walking with brief periods of jogging. The goal here is to add incrementally to your time spent jogging until ultimately it has replaced the walking altogether.

Here in San Jose, California, the city I have come to call home, it is possible to enjoy some form of outdoor activity virtually every day of the year. Wherever life finds you, make it impossible to use weather as an excuse for not being active. Your local sporting goods stores are well stocked with an array of home exercise devices that allow you to exert yourself from the comfort of your living room, basement, or den. Whatever your favorite video programs might be, know that they are no less funny, dramatic or suspenseful from the seat of a stationary bike or from the deck of a treadmill.

The important point with respect to stationary trainers is to put them front and center, place them in a location where they cannot be forgotten. I have witnessed far too often the sometimes subtle and other times not-so-subtle movements of these devices within homes.

It all begins innocently enough; the device is purchased with the best of intentions. One or more members of the family commit to using it thirty minutes a day, after all who among us can't find thirty minutes to invest in our good health. And for some all too brief stretch of time they do, until the neighbors are invited over for dinner. Not wanting the living room to look like a Gold's Gym, the equipment is pushed back into a spare bedroom. Two weeks later, the in-laws are in town and the exercise equipment goes out into the garage. Before its impressions have left the carpet, everything that could not otherwise find a home, has been piled onto it until some months later during the annual spring-cleaning it is all moved into the yard. There, for a small fraction of its original cost, the equipment is sold as part of a multifamily garage sale and the cycle begins anew. Heed my warning; do not allow your home exercise device to suffer a similar fate. Use the thing to its best purpose. Turn that investment in dollars into a return of pounds lost.

If your Manhattan loft is not of sufficient size or if your living arrangements are otherwise not conducive to the installation of home exercise equipment, you may want to consider a gym membership, a dispiriting notion to be sure. For many, but particularly for those who have little experience with exercise, the idea of doing so in a facility packed with people assumed to have more experience and therefore greater comfort is troubling. If that thought doesn't leave you feeling uneasy, the prospect of being made to interact with one of the club's membership consultants is sure to. These car salesmen in gym shorts will introduce you to various levels of membership and the fees associated with each. They will speak with you about the club's one-time or annual membership fees, processing fees, initiation fees, and periodic membership dues. If by the end of that conversation you haven't pulled all the hair out of your head, you will have proven your mettle and demonstrated the inner strength you'll need to survive in this alternate universe known as the commercial gym.

Truly, if you're unfamiliar with gyms and the denizens who populate them, then working out there is sure to be a unique experience. If exerting yourself in the presence of people who strain and struggle, grunt and groan to perform that final repetition makes you uncomfortable, if toweling-down a machine to remove someone else's sweat prior to your use leaves you queasy, if being asked to spot a guy as he prepares to bench press an amount of weight that would require a calculator to determine causes you to blanch, it is prudent to select carefully when choosing your gym.

Dependent upon the area in which you live, there may be several such gyms from which to choose. If you have a choice, choose wisely as that choice is sure to influence your willingness to use the gym on a consistent basis.

It is with the knowledge that many members will lose interest overtime that some gyms oversell their memberships. Don't surrender to self-doubt. Don't allow your commitment to yourself to wane. Once you have left your money and some measure of your perspiration at your gym of choice, be resolute in the task you have undertaken; you deserve success, you owe it to yourself. If you have met the challenges placed before you in this book, you have taken significant steps toward the completion of your journey. However far along that path you may have progressed, don't lose sight of your goal. While continuing your exercise program at a gym may be on some level annoying, try to think of it as a tool to be utilized or as a means to an end. Who knows, in time you may come to enjoy it. If not, use it only so long as necessary, and when the weather or other circumstances in your life allow, take your activity back outdoors.

In the interim, why not expose yourself to some of the other exercise activities to which your gym membership gives you access. You've paid your money, so shouldn't you get the most for it? From boxing to yoga, Pilates to tai chi and beyond, many clubs offer a wide variety of classes intended to address the varying needs and fitness levels of their clientele. Perhaps in one or more of them you will find an activity that kindles a passion for movement. Somewhere a tiny spark is waiting to ignite. Maybe you never imagined that you would find inspiration at a gym but why not there. I'm dating myself (as if I hadn't already done so with the Simon & Garfunkel reference) when I say that I used to find motivation in the workout scenes from the *Rocky* film series. Today, those scenes have been condensed and are available on *YouTube*. I don't mention it to encourage you to view them; my point is that inspiration can be found in the most unexpected places. I don't know that a gym would be considered an unexpected place to find such inspiration, but for one who had no interest in going to a gym let alone becoming a member, I think it is fair to refer to it as an unexpected place.

Clearly, the gym of today is a place far different from that in business even twenty years ago. The modern gym attempts to make a broader appeal and from a business perspective appropriately so. It's a poor business model that seeks to entice only the smallest percentage of the population. Success in the health and fitness industry today requires clubs provide a more all-encompassing approach to the creation of member services.

Despite that new orientation, weight equipment continues to occupy a significant percentage of most gym's floor space. This speaks to the fact that a good many members avail themselves of the ancient art of weight training. Performed primarily to strengthen our muscles, weight training also assists us in burning through the stored fat that for too many of us covers the musculature that through our gym memberships we're working so diligently to give shape to. In a misguided attempt to do away with fat, legions of exercisers complete their weight sessions with some period of time spent trying to crunch their way to six-pack abs. Sadly, that effort will leave those folks unfulfilled. One can do crunches until they're blue in the face and still fail to reveal that most cherished muscle formation.

From an anatomic perspective, I can tell you we all come equipped with that six-pack, exposing it, however, is not so much a function of crunches or any other abdominal exercise for that matter. It is most often the result of strict dieting and intense aerobic exercise. Still, if you entertain thoughts of yourself strolling along the beach with your washboard abdomen exposed for the world to see, options do exist. You can either have them painted on as some in Hollywood do, or you can do the hard work to rid yourself of those stored calories in hopes of unveiling them. Or you can simply accept the fact that but for a small percentage of the population, achieving the described abdomen is an unrealistic goal, and instead set your sights on decreasing your fat stores to become a healthier you.

Whatever the plans may be for your tummy, I would not discourage you from attempting to strengthen any part of your muscular anatomy, most especially the abdominal muscles. When properly attended, these muscles play an important role in maintaining our upright posture, are critical to the health of our backs and work to preserve the positioning of the organs that lie deep to them.

Interesting though these roles may be, I suspect most of us are inclined to think of them in a purely aesthetic sense. In that sense, our abdomens become our personal front porch. They are a reflection of the care and attention we invest in ourselves. In the same way a well-kept lawn provides curb appeal to our homes, a trim waistline does likewise for our bodies.

Whether it is form or function that stirs you to action, the paired goals of strengthening your abdomen and peeling away the fat that obscures it are laudable. Like weight loss itself though, these are time-intensive tasks. They will require sustained effort on both the exercise and calorie control fronts. This is not to say that it can't be done but that it will require patience and persistence. Patience, we're told, is a virtue. Within the context of remodeling your physical self, having patience is especially virtuous. Throughout the course of this book, its presence has been alluded to, although not always expressly. Here, the Chinese proverb that roughly translates to a journey of a thousand miles begins with a single step, seems especially apropos. However long, difficult, or challenging a particular task might be, the road to its completion begins by taking that first measured step. The proverb speaks rather generally to the idea of getting started, but it also implies a need for patience and perseverance to see a venture through to its conclusion.

By purchasing this book, you have taken your first step, and dependent upon the degree to which you have implemented its recommendations, perhaps you've taken many more. Regardless their number, your steps are the undertaking of a person determined to bring change to your life. You are the artist, your body is your medium, create your masterpiece.

Chapter 14

Lessons from Beyond the World of Weight Loss

From the outset, I have written of the difficulties attendant to weight loss. It has not been my intention to discourage but to make plain it is a tall hurdle for us all. Perhaps in your prior experience you have already come to know what a formidable foe excess weight can be. Regardless your personal history with it, the statistics concerning weight loss suggest each of us who confront it will wage many wars in an effort to win victory. Yet victory over our weight remains elusive.

Although surely not referencing weight loss, Proverbs 24:6 advises that war not be waged in the absence of sound counsel, and that only through the advice of many counselors can a war be won. Without getting into the real-world military implications of the passage, I will agree that more information is generally better. However, when the information presented is contradictory, what then? As it pertains to our weight, each of us who square off against it becomes our own final arbiter. Taking counsel in this regard is appropriate, but as is true with war itself, the decision to proceed or not ultimately rests with one. In this one particular war through which you aim to reduce your weight, do you hand over authority to others, or do you subscribe to the view that success in this matter will not come from the efforts of others, but rather from your own dogged determination?

In her book *Lean In*, author and business leader Sheryl Sandberg addresses women in the workplace. She calls upon them to reject the fear that prevents them from pursuing, in no particular order, professional success, and personal fulfillment. To illustrate her point, Sandberg recalls the feelings of angst she experienced while driving to a new job. She anticipated the job would be difficult and was uncertain of her ability to meet its challenges. She recounts the moments when she didn't believe in herself; convinced only of her own inadequacy, she was certain that in every task and in every job she would fail. From her own feelings of impotence, Sandberg recognized a pattern of behavior that she discovered was not unique to her. Other women, she learned, took the same halting steps designed less to achieve success than to eschew it.

Like the biblical reference, Sandberg is not addressing weight loss in her tome, but with her sentiments, she could just as easily do so. Whatever else weight loss may be, it is certainly a battle, one fought in large measure in our minds; a clash between our desire to overcome it and the absence of the belief needed to achieve it. Were Sandburg herself to advise you on the subject, I'm sure she would exhort you, as she does women bent on ascending the corporate ladder - to lean in, to take action, to believe in yourself, and to believe in your dreams. In her stead, I will encourage you to break the bonds of fear that to this point have made weight loss at best a fleeting success.

In chapter 2, I referred to our propensity to undermine our efforts to achieve success in the area of weight loss. Be aware these efforts to undermine are not limited to our desire to lose weight. A good many of us, men and women alike, cannot bear to see ourselves succeed at any venture. In our careers, in our interpersonal relationships, in our lives in general, we unconsciously create impediments to achieving the goals we consciously seek.

Those who know me would sarcastically say I am a great one to offer up this wisdom. They would tell you where negative thinking is concerned I am the exemplar. I would argue that as one who has long suffered from the consequences of self-doubt, there might be no single person who could speak more earnestly on the subject than I can. Looking back, I can point to examples in my own life where I have passed on opportunities that might have yielded greater personal happiness or professional success. Through the filter of hindsight, I now recognize that for me the fear of the unknown, of being shaken out of the small but stable life I had created for myself, acted as an anchor. It prevented me, in the same way an anchor would, of reaching beyond the life I knew to the life I had long before only imagined.

I do not occupy the rank or social standing I had so long ago coveted. During the course of my lifetime, I have repeatedly acted as my own worst enemy. To the extent that I had known any success in my life, I convinced myself it would not carry over to the next level. In the darker recesses of my mind, I knew if I had accepted the opportunities offered to me, I would ultimately be found out and exposed as an imposter. Rather than inviting success, I anticipated failure. As a result I, like Sheryl Sandberg and countless others, leaned back when opportunities were extended.

Unfortunately, as a child, I didn't realize that reaching for the brass ring on the merry-go-round was a metaphor for life. To be successful at any pursuit, we must reach out beyond our arm's length. We must extend ourselves and in so doing step outside of our comfort zone.

Yes, on a conscious level we all want the trappings of success to surround us. In our quieter moments, I believe we each imagine a life made better by the improved access to goods and services made possible by greater success in our chosen fields of endeavor. While we may wish for it, we are paralyzed in our actions to achieve it. With our glass is bone-dry attitude, we throw our energy into examining the negative fallout of this hoped-for success.

As it pertains to our weight, rather than giving thought to the positive change that shedding pounds would bring to our lives, we instead worry about how it might adversely affect us. We fear the weight loss would alter the perceptions of people close to us about who we are. We worry it may in fact alter how we think about ourselves, causing us to lose our identity. We fear that the friends who had embraced the fuller bodied us might reject the leaner version of ourselves. We experience anxiety that with these changes come unsustainable changes to our lifestyles and our lives in general.

In our minds, the scenario more likely to play out finds us failing (yet again) to achieve our weight loss goals and disappointing those around us. Even if we were to succeed on the short term, we convince ourselves that the weight would soon enough find its way back to us, and the disappointment registering on the faces of friends and family members would be all the greater. Given all the imagined negatives that could grow out of our attempts to achieve some measure of success in our lives, it is a wonder any of us would dare to step outside the house. However, in our self-imposed confinement, all that we hope to achieve will always exist as dreams unfulfilled.

No one, least of all me, would be so bold as to suggest that calling attention to a problem, whatever that problem may be, is enough to conquer it. Still, we must first be aware of the existence of a problem before we can institute the measures needed to overcome it. Does a fear of success hold you back? Has the joy that comes from having accomplished a personal or professional goal thus far eluded you? If so, examine your fears and determine whether your reasons for them stand up to careful scrutiny.

As it applies to your weight, I think you will find most of your fears won't hold water. Your friends who are truly your friends, would never abandon you over a goal that you set out to achieve. Friends by definition are those people who support you through all of your exertions, but particularly through those that lead to a more healthy and vibrant you.

Regardless its exact nature, if fear restrains you, know that it is an especially unrelenting nemesis. Fear confounds us and leaves us blind to the opportunities at hand. I recall an occasion when I had gone rock climbing with a couple of friends in Yosemite Valley. I had fallen back a touch when I came upon what appeared to me to be a smooth granite surface. In my mind, the rock had more the appearance of a sheet of glass than something that had been shaped by nature. On it, I could find no hand or footholds that would allow me to advance up the formation. Even though I knew both of my climbing partners had ascended the same rock, I could not envision how they had done so. Finding no means by which I could pull myself up, I shouted, "I've got nothing". Following a brief and disquieting period of laughter they told to look again because the holds were there. Armed with the reassurance of my friends, I found those holds and sometime later enjoyed a view of one of the most beautiful places on the planet, a view that a relatively few have seen, or will ever see.

With the help of my friends, I put aside the fear that had clouded my vision and in the end, I was rewarded for doing so. My prize was to see what Theodore Roosevelt referred to as "a great solemn cathedral, far vaster and more beautiful than any built by the hand of man". For a far too brief period, I savored my reward as we soon thereafter descended back to the valley floor. The reward that lies in store for you, however, need not be constrained by time. Once you have met your weight loss goal, it can be yours to hold onto and relish. If fear impedes you in this purpose, work to cast it off, and be done with it. Overcome the trepidation that to this point has made it impossible for you to achieve this very worthwhile goal, and then bask in the satisfaction that comes from having achieved it.

Chapter 15

The AMA Weighs In

On the very day I completed my manuscript the American Medical Association (AMA) stepped forward to declare that obesity was a disease. As part of a press release tied to that announcement, AMA board member Patrice Harris, MD claimed that "recognizing obesity as a disease will help change the way the medical community tackles this complex issue that affects approximately one in three Americans". Dr. Harris went on to say, "The AMA is committed to improving health outcomes and is working to reduce the incidence of cardiovascular disease and type 2 diabetes, which are often linked to obesity."

Although it is far too early to know what affect their newly adopted position will have on the treatment of obesity in this country, I would like to take this opportunity to share my thoughts on how I believe this is likely to shake out. Remembering that I am neither a physician nor a fortuneteller, my thoughts may be mine alone, but my advice would be to follow the money.

Another credential I do not possess is that of a financial consultant. Still, if you were looking to profit from the fact that obesity has been elevated to a disease status, I would tell you to look past the many companies that churn out supplements purported to aid in weight loss. Because many of these companies are privately held and not publically traded, they will be content to keep the money they make for themselves. Regardless, look for them to alter their marketing to reflect the AMA's new stance. I can see their advertisements now. Either they buy a physician to speak about the virtues of their new and improved formulations, or they hire someone from central casting, give him a white lab coat, and a pair of glasses (to affect a scholarly and paternal vibe). He will speak in soothing and conciliatory tones about the utter hopelessness of this disease, which only now, through the intervention of their proprietary blend of encapsulated ingredients like polio before it, can be conquered.

Better options from an investment perspective might be the pharmaceutical companies that will put more of their own money behind efforts to develop and bring to market new drugs to fight obesity. Alternatively, consider researching those companies that manufacture bariatric surgical instruments and related appliances, since accepting the disease model is likely to result in an increase in the number of gastric bypasses performed.

Call it a disease if you prefer, but I remain steadfast in my belief that neither pills nor surgery offers the best solution, because the underlying issue of disordered eating and our pathologic relationship with food are not being addressed. With regard to the surgical procedures in particular, they not only fail to speak to the issues related to our maladaptive feeding behaviors, they in some ways perpetuate them.

The anatomical changes brought about by these surgeries require that the patient make radical alterations in the proportion, composition, and even pace of their meals. But do the anatomical changes themselves *force* the alteration in eating habits or must the patient still make the choice to change?

According to one study published in *Psychology and Health* (Negotiating control: Patients' experiences of unsuccessful weight loss surgery, Ogden, Avenell, et al, Vol. 26, No. 7, July 2011, 949-964), among patients who claimed that their procedures failed to produce the desired outcome, namely significant weight loss, all believed that the failure was at least in part the result of the lack of attention given to the mental/emotional aspects of weight loss.

In discussing the reasons for the failure as they perceived them, some patients alleged the restricted stomach capacity brought about by the surgery did not sufficiently limit or control what or how much they ate. Clearly, what they had hoped for was that their new anatomy would hold sway over their eating, that they could effectively give control over to their surgically altered anatomy, and in effect become passive partners in the weight loss process.

Blaming the surgery may be unfair and perhaps even maladaptive, especially when combined with the patients' reports of having discovered ways in which they could, in a matter of speaking, cheat the system. Rather than adhering to the strict dietary guidelines, some patients developed strategies that enabled them to eat more freely. According to one patient, "I found that if I chewed the food tremendously to a pulp I could actually get more of it, quite frequently....I actually ate anything I felt like eating."

While I have to say that this is but one small study, it is interesting to note the continuation of disordered eating reported, despite a surgical treatment intended to prevent it. Supporting these findings are additional studies that indicate poorer weight loss outcomes among patients who struggle to comply with the postoperative eating guidelines and research that revealed continued dysfunctional eating behaviors including emotional eating and grazing, defined as a pattern of behavior in which one repeatedly consumes smaller quantities of food during a protracted period of time.

It is understood that obesity is a multi-layered issue and intrinsic to it are both medical and psychological factors. In its extreme state, obesity places its sufferers in imminent peril, and when confronted with such circumstances, it may be necessary to undertake drastic measures. As it pertains to weight loss, there can be no more drastic measure than gastric bypass. Performing this procedure presupposes that A) despite efforts made to curb the maladaptive behaviors that lead to the weight gain, the individual is either unwilling or for some other reason unable to commit to the changes needed to bring about the required weight loss. Stated another way, all of the noninvasive alternatives have been exhausted; and B) the weight gain is so severe and the associated health consequences so profound that other options have been ruled out or simply don't exist.

Even with these conditions met, bariatric surgery is not a procedure to be taken lightly. On both the plus and minus sides, it is likely to be a life altering procedure. While I will make no effort to dispute its efficacy in the treatment of the morbidly obese, I can't help but have my reservations about the procedure in general. With all due respect, to the physicians who developed the procedure and all who perform it, I must say that when you're a hammer, everything looks like a nail.

As the expression applies to surgeons, when confronted with a problem, look for them to find solutions through surgery. This is not meant to be a dig at surgeons. It is, I think, a natural tendency to employ one's own unique skill set when attempting to tackle a problem. Within this context, it is fair for bariatric surgeons to find their answers to obesity through the surgical treatment of the stomach. However, since the stomach is technically not the problem, is the surgical treatment of it the answer?

The question brings to mind a conversation I had with a physician friend of mine several years ago. We were discussing surgical options for the treatment of a knee injury sustained by an athlete under my charge. When discussing one of the options, the physician, an orthopedic surgeon, referred to it by saying that it amounted to "treating pathology with pathology", or put another way, the procedure in question treats disease by creating disease. I believe that bariatric surgeons are doing exactly that with the gastric bypass (and related procedures), although in its case what is being treated is at worst a mental/emotional pathology. The stomach, which in one form or another is the target of the surgeon's attention, is functioning as intended.

When addressing the issue of multivitamins I spoke about the arrogance of man. In that instance, I suggested that it was our collective sense of self-importance that allows us to believe we are capable of improving upon nature's gifts.

I raise that same concern in connection to bariatric surgery. I have long been astonished by the human organism, that thin or thick, fit or fat we are each an engineering marvel. Complete as equipped, in a perfect world we have no need of augmentation, alteration, or enhancement.

Unfortunately, for some of us, the circumstances of our lives at times dictate the need for augmentation or alteration. When life requires such treatment, the anatomical changes created by it may give rise to some unintended physiologic effects. As it applies to bariatric surgery, the effects may be many and varied. To those who have entertained the thought of such a procedure, I encourage you to not only know, but also understand the consequences, and then ask yourself this very important question: am I truly incapable of losing weight through conventional means? If you answer in the affirmative, perhaps a bariatric procedure is right for you. If, on the other hand, any part of you believes that you can overcome this challenge through means other than surgery, then I urge you to give it your full effort.

For the purpose of clarity, let me again state that I am not a physician, and in the area of bariatric surgery, I claim no special expertise, but I can't help but wonder what history will ultimately teach us about the procedure. When blessed with the benefit of hindsight, will we look back upon the surgery as the option of best choice when dealing with obesity or will we see it as a primitive and misguided attempt to surgically address a complex eating disorder? In this matter, I hope the bariatric surgeons prove to be more prescient than I am. A Californian born and raised, I had the foresight and good sense to take French when attending high school in the seventies never imagining that Spanish might prove to be more useful.

Whatever the truth proves to be, it will surely be borne out in time. Until then, of one thing I am absolutely certain, we must intervene far earlier in our efforts to address disordered eating, long before the hole has been dug so deep that it is no longer possible to climb out without assistance. Being obese is not something we aspire to, it is instead a manifestation of disordered eating that may itself grow out of other deep-seated psychosocial issues. As in most other problems in our lives, our issues related to eating are best dealt with before they have taken root.

Chapter 16

Closing Arguments

With the dawning of each new day, we are all made to face tests and challenges. It is, I suppose, the nature of our existence to meet, confront, take on, beat back, and when possible, win victory over our troubles. We can face and dispense with some of the issues in relatively short order: work assignments, some interpersonal issues, even some financial matters need not necessarily linger long. In these matters, one can often find final resolution by a date certain, but not so our difficulties with weight. There exists no specific period within which we can shed ten or twenty pounds. The rate at which we lose weight, or for that matter gain it, is tied directly to our energy (read as calorie) surplus or deficit. How we achieve that deficit (since it is the primary purpose of this book is to assist you in losing weight; gaining weight is not a problem with which most of us struggle) is a function of the separate but related roles of energy intake and output. Simple matters really, were it not for the countless landmines that life puts in our paths. We promise to take steps toward reducing our food intake, but we apply conditions. We will do so after the holidays, or following our vacation, or on the first of the month, which invariably becomes the first of the following month, and the following month, and the following month, ad infinitum.

So too our commitment to embrace exercise, but with similar conditions and escape clauses, we provide ourselves with excuses that allow us to push back, delay, and inevitably avoid the exertions. Still, the thought of weight loss, if not the actions that presuppose it, stay with us. We want it, we wish for it, and yet when it comes time for the rubber to meet the road, we balk.

Perhaps that too is in our nature, to avoid those things that are difficult, opting instead to do that which supplies the least resistance, which we can accomplish with the smallest of efforts. After all, isn't it easier to simply buy the next size up in the garment of your choice than to do the work that achieves weight loss? Isn't it easier to continue as we have rather than alter our actions for the purpose of losing weight? We can easily do these things to avoid the hard work of weight loss.

If you thought you would find an easy solution to weight loss when you purchased this book, I'm afraid I have disappointed you. Although to be fair, I made it clear from the outset that weight loss is nothing of the sort. Throughout the preceding pages, I have worked to impress upon you the grueling and sometimes cruel nature of weight loss and to dispel the notion that easy and/or quick solutions exist. Yet the promises of rapid weight loss made by others are stated with equal conviction, leaving you, as before, ever hopeful.

Possessed of that hope as you may be, I believe that you still intuitively know you cannot accomplish weight loss without struggle. In my efforts to assist you in this process, I have attempted to make that abundantly clear. If the path that led you to your present weight was easily trod, the path back is likely to be perceived as uphill all the way. As you now stand at the base of that hill, you are most likely questioning, as you probably have in the past, your ability to reach the summit. However, if weight loss is to be more than a wish, a hope, a dream, you must take appropriate actions. If you truly mean for it to switch sides of the ledger, to go from being something you hoped to achieve to something you have achieved, if it is not merely idle chatter but sincere desire that compels you to act then act boldly, be purposeful in your quest. You've bought the book and presumably, you have read it, unless of course, you've treated it like a Dan Brown novel and jumped ahead to the end in order to learn the identity of the responsible party. However, in this *who done it* you are the responsible party.

If after having taken the measure of the message you believe the path I propose is sustainable, then begin your journey, or if your journey has already begun, please carry on. Yes, without question, you will need to make sacrifices. At the very least, it will be necessary to take stock of the foods you do eat and decrease the presence of the calorie-dense items in your diet. It has been my position all along that one need not eliminate those foods, but they must be less frequently featured, and on those occasions when they do find their way onto your plate, they should play a supporting role to foods of greater nutrient density and lesser calorie cost. This is a critical concept because we want to and need to enjoy the foods we eat, but at the same time, we cannot lose sight of the fact that they are primarily sources of energy. As such, we should exercise more discretion when determining what and how much we eat.

Still, I can't expect you to alter completely the eating habits that you've established during the course of your lifetime. My objective has been to nudge you in the direction of better food choices believing that through that nudging your ties to more calorie-laden foods will erode in time. Sadly, what I believe means nothing if you yourself do not. To achieve success, you must first believe in the process and in your ability to see it through. While it may not be possible for us to accomplish *everything* we set our minds to, what is certainly true is that we cannot accomplish *anything* if we neither believe in it nor commit ourselves to it. Here I don't ask for your commitment. Rather I ask *you* to ask it of yourself.

As I have said repeatedly, the task before you is difficult, but greater feats have been achieved. For those among you who have fought this battle in fits and starts over the span of many years, perhaps there is no greater feat than to establish or reestablish control over your weight. Doing so will not occur as a function of luck. Luck can serve you in your profession, in your daily life, even in love, but as it applies to weight loss, luck plays no role. The degree to which you know success will be a direct result of your own efforts. Call upon friends and family members to support you if you need, physicians and other healthcare providers to guide you if you like, but at the end of the day, the work is yours to do. Through it, you will not be changing society's attitudes toward eating, our goal is to change yours.

As a society, we will continue to celebrate nutritional perversities. Rather than applauding those who lose weight for the sake of their own good health, we appear to prefer rewarding those who demonstrate excellence in the area of gluttony. Celebrity status has been conferred upon Joey Chestnut and Takeru Kobayashi and their peers for doing nothing more than eating massive quantities of food. The exploits of these competitive eaters have been broadcast for the world to see on sports-programming networks. Competitive though their contests may be, those who participate could not by any stretch of the imagination be thought of as sportsmen, nor, consequently, should their events be elevated or made credible by being telecast for international, national, or even local audiences. To my way of thinking, such contests are circus acts that take disordered eating to preposterous levels. The very idea of eating sixty-two hotdogs in ten minutes time is insane on the face of it. In fact, the accomplishment of eating sixty-two anything in such a brief span of time is an act more suitable for revulsion than praise. More revolting still is what becomes of those meals at the end of the contest. Although never discussed, one would have to believe, based upon the physiques of the most successful gourmands, the events are followed by some period of purging.

Dental decay and upper GI tract erosions aside, the life of a celebrity binge eater might appear alluring - all the food you can hold down and prize money to boot. While I would like to think that no one would be drawn to such pursuits, there may be no limits to which some will go to achieve a measure of fame. For that reason primarily, I would advise those who see fit to broadcast this nonsense to include a discussion of how the contestants prepare for an event, and how they spend their time in the minutes, hours, and days following the event, and then stand it up against proper nutritional practices. Broadcasters may argue that, like the Houston Rodeo, they are not in business to educate, to which I would say by making such programming available they do tacitly condone it, and unless they would want that to be the perception, they should provide a counterpoint.

A counterpoint to disordered eating is what I have championed throughout this book. Unfortunately, my reach is limited. With more than eighty thousand competing titles in print, I would be naïve to believe that my thoughts will turn the tide in our country's slide toward ever-greater numbers of overweight or obese men, women, and children. After all, mine is just another voice in the crowd. Still, I'd like to think some will hear my message and be moved to take on the challenge. I cannot promise, as others have, that by doing so you will extend your life. There are simply too many intervening variables to make such a claim. However, I do believe that by attaining and maintaining an appropriate weight, you can live the years you do have in as healthy a fashion as possible, free from the fear and regret that for too long has stifled your ability to live your dreams.

The 12 Keys to Achieving Your Weight Loss Goals

1. Be dogged in your determination. Expect to succeed!
2. Don't allow short-term setbacks to derail your efforts to achieve your long-term goals.
3. Work to reduce the presence of foods that are low in nutrient value and high in saturated fat from your diet.
4. Bring color to your diet by increasing your consumption of fruits and vegetables.
5. Expose more of your plate by eating smaller portions.
6. Find room in your life for activity.
7. Redefine your lifestyle by subtracting out the modern conveniences that have made movement less necessary.
8. Limit your intake of "liquid calories", particularly those coming in the form of alcohol and soft drinks.
9. Be aware of your numbers but not obsessed with them. Know your approximate calorie consumption but don't be distracted by weights and measures.

10. Know why you're eating what you're eating; make an effort to eat for the purpose of satisfying hunger.
11. Avoid eating within 2 hours of your bedtime, not because the body processes the calories differently, but because these are frequently calories of habit and not hunger.
12. Seek out the support of others if need be, but ultimately you must rely upon yourself. This task is yours to accomplish!